LOW CARB

RECIPES

COOKBOOK

Guide to Simple and Wholesome Meals for Overall Health

JENNIFER STEWART

TABLE OF CONTENTS

INTRODUCTION TO THE LOW-CARB LIFESTYLE

The low-carb lifestyle is all about reducing the number of carbohydrates you consume daily. Instead of getting most of your calories from carbs like bread, pasta, and sugary foods, you focus more on proteins, healthy fats, and vegetables. This approach helps stabilize blood sugar levels, curb cravings, and promote overall health.

Benefits of a Low-Carb Diet

1. Weight Loss

One of the most popular reasons people turn to a low-carb diet is for weight loss. By cutting down on carbs, your body starts burning fat for energy, which can lead to significant weight loss. Plus, you will often feel fuller longer, which means you are less likely to overeat.

2. Better Blood Sugar Control

For those with diabetes or insulin resistance, a low-carb diet can be a game-changer. Lowering carb intake helps prevent blood sugar spikes and crashes, leading to more stable energy levels throughout the day.

3. Improved Heart Health

A low-carb diet can also benefit your heart. It helps reduce levels of triglycerides (a type of fat in the blood), increase HDL (good cholesterol), and lower LDL (bad cholesterol), all of which contribute to better heart health.

4. Increased Energy Levels

Many people report feeling more energetic on a low-carb diet. Without the highs and lows caused by fluctuating blood sugar levels, you can enjoy steady energy throughout the day.

5. Enhanced Mental Clarity

Cutting down on carbs can also improve your mental clarity and focus. The brain can efficiently use ketones (produced when you eat fewer carbs) as a source of energy, which some find helps them think more clearly.

6. Reduced Cravings and Hunger

A low-carb diet often leads to reduced hunger and fewer cravings. Protein and fats are more satiating than carbs, helping you feel full and satisfied for longer periods.

7. Better Digestion

Many people experience better digestion on a low-carb diet. Reducing carb-heavy foods like bread and pasta can alleviate issues like bloating and gas.

By embracing a low-carb lifestyle, you're taking a significant step towards improving your overall health and well-being. This book is designed to make that journey easier and more enjoyable, offering you a wide range of delicious recipes and practical tips to sustain your new eating habits.

Common Myths and Misconceptions

When it comes to low-carb diets, there are several myths and misconceptions that can make it confusing or intimidating to start. Let's clear up some of the most common ones:

1. Myth: Low-Carb Diets Are Unhealthy

Fact: Some people believe that cutting out carbs means missing out on essential nutrients. However, a well-balanced low-carb diet includes plenty of vegetables, healthy fats, and high-quality proteins, providing all the nutrients your body needs. It's all about choosing the right kinds of foods.

2. Myth: You Can't Eat Any Carbs

Fact: A low-carb diet doesn't mean zero carbs. It simply means reducing your intake, especially from sources like refined sugars, bread, and pasta. You can still enjoy carbs from vegetables, nuts, seeds, and even some fruits, just in moderation.

3. Myth: Low-Carb Diets Are High in Unhealthy Fats

Fact: While low-carb diets do include fats, the focus is on healthy fats from sources like avocados, nuts, seeds, olive oil, and fatty fish. These fats are beneficial for heart health and overall well-being. It's all about choosing the right types of fats.

4. Myth: Low-Carb Diets Cause Nutrient Deficiencies

Fact: When done correctly, a low-carb diet is rich in nutrient-dense foods. You'll be eating a variety of vegetables, nuts, seeds, and high-quality proteins that provide essential vitamins and minerals. Nutrient deficiencies are unlikely if the diet is well-planned.

5. Myth: You'll Feel Tired All the Time

Fact: It's common to feel a bit sluggish during the first few days as your body adjusts, a phase often referred to as the "keto flu." However, once your body adapts to burning fat for fuel instead of carbs, many people report having more energy than before.

6. Myth: Low-Carb Diets Are Just a Fad

Fact: Low-carb diets have been around for a long time and are supported by a significant body of research. They have proven benefits for weight loss, blood sugar control, and overall health. Unlike fad diets, low-carb eating is sustainable and can be maintained long-term.

7. Myth: You Can't Exercise on a Low-Carb Diet

Fact: While it might take a little time for your body to adjust, many people successfully exercise and even thrive on a low-carb diet. Your body can use fat for fuel, which can sustain both endurance and strength activities. There are even professional athletes who follow low-carb diets.

8. Myth: All Carbs Are Bad

Fact: Not all carbs are created equal. Processed and refined carbs can lead to health issues, but complex carbs from vegetables and whole foods are beneficial. It's important to distinguish between the types of carbs you're consuming.

By understanding these myths and misconceptions, you can approach a low-carb diet with confidence, knowing that it's a healthy and effective way to improve your overall well-being. This book will guide you through the process, making it easier to adopt and maintain a low-carb lifestyle.

CHAPTER 1

Understanding the Low Carb Diet

What is a Low-Carb Diet?

A low-carb diet is a dietary approach that limits the intake of carbohydrates, typically found in sugary foods, pasta, and bread. Instead of relying on carbs for energy, a low-carb diet emphasizes the consumption of proteins, healthy fats, and vegetables. The primary goal is to shift the body's metabolism from burning glucose (a type of sugar) to burning fat for energy, a state known as ketosis.

Carbohydrates are a primary source of energy for the body, but when consumed in excess, they can lead to weight gain and various health issues like insulin resistance and type 2 diabetes. By reducing carb intake, you can help stabilize blood sugar levels, reduce hunger, and promote weight loss.

Different Types of Low-Carb Diets

There are several variations of low-carb diets, each with its unique approach and guidelines. Below are some of the most popular types:

1. Ketogenic (Keto) Diet

The ketogenic diet is a very low-carb, high-fat diet that aims to put your body into a state of ketosis. In ketosis, the body burns fat for energy instead of carbs.

Carb Intake: Typically limited to 20-50 grams per day.

Key Foods: High-fat foods like avocados, nuts, seeds, oils, fatty fish, and meats. Low-carb vegetables like leafy greens, broccoli, and cauliflower.

Benefits: Rapid weight loss, improved mental clarity, and better blood sugar control.

Challenges: Initial side effects known as the "keto flu" (headaches, fatigue, nausea), it requires strict adherence to maintain ketosis.

2. Atkins Diet

The Atkins diet is one of the most well-known low-carb diets, divided into four phases. It starts with very low carb intake and gradually increases the amount of allowed carbs.

Carb Intake: Starts with 20 grams per day during the induction phase, gradually increasing in subsequent phases.

Key Foods: Meat, fish, eggs, cheese, fats, low-carb vegetables, and later, nuts, seeds, and berries.

Benefits: Effective for weight loss and improving metabolic health, flexible after the initial phase.

Challenges: Can be restrictive during the initial phase, potential for nutrient deficiencies if not well-balanced.

3. Paleo Diet

The Paleo diet focuses on eating whole, unprocessed foods similar to what our ancestors might have eaten. It emphasizes lean proteins, fruits, vegetables, nuts, and seeds while avoiding processed foods, grains, legumes, and dairy.

Carb Intake: Generally low to moderate, depending on the individual's food choices.

Key Foods: Grass-fed meat, fish, eggs, vegetables, fruits, nuts, and seeds.

Benefits: Emphasis on whole foods, improved digestion, weight loss, and better blood sugar control.

Challenges: Can be challenging to follow strictly, potential social and lifestyle adjustments, may require careful planning to ensure nutritional balance.

4. Low-Carb, High-Fat (LCHF) Diet

Similar to the ketogenic diet but slightly less restrictive. Focuses on reducing carbs and increasing healthy fat intake.

Carb Intake: Typically under 100 grams per day, but can vary.

Key Foods: High-fat foods like oils, butter, fatty fish, and avocados, along with moderate protein and low-carb vegetables.

Benefits: Weight loss, improved satiety, better blood sugar control.

Challenges: Adjusting to higher fat intake, potential need for monitoring fat quality.

5. Whole30

Whole30 is a 30-day elimination diet that focuses on whole foods and eliminates sugar, alcohol, grains, legumes, soy, and dairy. After 30 days, foods are reintroduced one at a time to identify any potential food sensitivities.

Carb Intake: Low to moderate, depending on individual choices.

Key Foods: Meat, seafood, eggs, vegetables, fruits, and natural fats.

Benefits: It helps identify food sensitivities, promotes whole food consumption, and aids in weight loss.

Challenges: Highly restrictive, significant planning and preparation required, social and dining out challenges.

Each of these low-carb diets has its unique benefits and challenges, and the best one for you will depend on your personal health goals, lifestyle, and preferences. By understanding these different approaches, you can choose the one that fits your needs and helps you achieve your health and wellness objectives.

How to Determine Your Ideal Carb Intake

Determining the ideal amount of carbohydrates for your diet can be a personalized process, as it depends on various factors such as your health goals, activity level, and metabolic health. Here's a step-by-step guide to help you find the right balance:

Step 1: Define Your Goals

Identify your primary reason for adopting a low-carb diet. Common goals include:

- **Weight Loss:** To promote fat burning and weight loss, a lower carb intake might be necessary.
- **Blood Sugar Control:** Managing conditions like diabetes or insulin resistance may require stricter carb limits.
- **Improved Energy Levels:** Balancing carbs to maintain stable energy throughout the day.

Step 2: Understand Carb Categories

Carbohydrates come in different forms, with varying impacts on blood sugar levels. Understanding these can help you make better choices:

- **Simple Carbs:** Found in sugary foods and drinks, these cause quick spikes in blood sugar and are best minimized.
- **Complex Carbs:** Found in whole grains, legumes, and vegetables, these digest more slowly and have a gentler effect on blood sugar.

Step 3: Start with a General Guideline

Begin with a common low-carb range and adjust based on your body's response:

- **Very Low-Carb/Ketogenic:** 20-50 grams of net carbs per day. Ideal for rapid weight loss and achieving ketosis.
- **Moderate Low-Carb:** 50-100 grams of net carbs per day. Suitable for steady weight loss, better blood sugar control, and improved energy.

- **Liberal Low-Carb:** 100-150 grams of net carbs per day. Good for maintaining weight and general health without strict restrictions.

Net carbs are calculated by subtracting fiber and sugar alcohols from the total carbs, as these do not significantly impact blood sugar.

Step 4: Track and Adjust

Track your daily carb intake using a food diary or a mobile app. Monitor your body's response, including:

- **Weight Changes:** Weekly weight tracking can indicate if your carb intake is supporting your weight loss goals.
- **Energy Levels:** Note how your energy fluctuates throughout the day. Adjust your carb intake to avoid energy crashes.
- **Hunger and Cravings:** Pay attention to your hunger levels and cravings. If you're constantly hungry, you might need to adjust your carb or protein intake.

Step 5: Consider Your Activity Level

Active individuals, especially those engaging in high-intensity workouts, might need more carbs for optimal performance. Adjust your intake to match your energy expenditure:

- **Sedentary Lifestyle:** Lower end of the carb spectrum (20-50 grams).
- **Moderately Active:** Moderate intake (50-100 grams).
- **Highly Active:** Higher intake, still within low-carb limits (100-150 grams).

Transitioning to a Low-Carb Lifestyle

Transitioning to a low-carb lifestyle can be smooth and sustainable with the right approach. Here are some tips to help you make the shift:

1. Gradual Reduction

If you're accustomed to a high-carb diet, consider gradually reducing your carb intake over a few weeks. This approach can help minimize withdrawal symptoms and make the transition more manageable.

2. Focus on Whole Foods

Base your diet on whole, unprocessed foods like vegetables, meats, fish, eggs, nuts, and seeds. Avoid processed and refined carbs, which can lead to cravings and energy spikes.

3. Stay Hydrated

Drinking plenty of water is essential, especially during the initial phase. Adequate hydration helps your body adapt to the changes and can alleviate common side effects like headaches and fatigue.

4. Balance Your Macros

Ensure your meals are balanced with proteins, healthy fats, and low-carb vegetables. This balance helps keep you full and satisfied, reducing the likelihood of cravings and overeating.

5. Plan and Prepare Meals

Meal planning and preparation are key to staying on track. Having low-carb meals and snacks readily available can prevent you from reaching for high-carb options when hunger strikes.

6. Monitor Your Progress

Keep track of your weight, energy levels, and overall well-being. Use this information to adjust your carb intake and food choices as needed to meet your goals.

7. Stay Consistent

Consistency is crucial for long-term success. Stick to your low-carb plan, even on weekends and holidays, to maintain progress and avoid setbacks.

8. Seek Support

Join a community or find a support group, either online or in-person, to share experiences, tips, and encouragement. Having a support network can make the transition easier and more enjoyable.

By determining your ideal carb intake and following these steps to transition smoothly, you can successfully adopt a low-carb lifestyle and enjoy its numerous health benefits.

CHAPTER 2

Essential Low Carb Foods

Stocking your kitchen with the right low-carb foods is important for making the transition easier and maintaining a low-carb lifestyle. The following is a comprehensive guide to essential low-carb foods, including pantry staples, fresh produce and proteins, healthy fats and oils, sweeteners and condiments, and ingredient substitutions.

Pantry Staples

Keeping your pantry stocked with low-carb essentials ensures you always have the ingredients needed to prepare quick and healthy meals. Here are some must-haves:

- **Nuts and Seeds:** Almonds, walnuts, chia seeds, flaxseeds, and pumpkin seeds.
- **Nut Butters:** Almond butter, peanut butter (unsweetened), and sunflower seed butter.
- **Low-Carb Flours:** Almond flour, coconut flour, and flaxseed meal.
- **Canned Goods:** Tuna, salmon, sardines, and chicken in water or olive oil.
- **Broth/Stock:** Chicken, beef, and vegetable broth (low-sodium preferred).
- **Coconut Products:** Coconut milk, coconut cream, and unsweetened shredded coconut.

- **Spices and Herbs:** Basil, oregano, thyme, paprika, cumin, garlic powder, onion powder, and turmeric.
- **Olives and Pickles:** Low-carb and sugar-free varieties.

Fresh Produce and Proteins

A variety of fresh vegetables and high-quality proteins are the foundation of a healthy low-carb diet. Stock up on these items:

- **Vegetables:** Leafy greens (spinach, kale, arugula), cruciferous vegetables (broccoli, cauliflower, Brussels sprouts), zucchini, bell peppers, asparagus, cucumber, and mushrooms.
- **Berries:** Strawberries, blueberries, raspberries, and blackberries (in moderation).
- **Proteins:**
  - ★ **Meat and Poultry:** Chicken, turkey, beef, pork, and lamb.
  - ★ **Fish and Seafood:** Salmon, mackerel, sardines, shrimp, and crab.
  - ★ **Eggs:** A versatile protein source, always keep plenty on hand.
- **Dairy:** Cheese (cheddar, mozzarella, feta), full-fat Greek yogurt (unsweetened), and heavy cream.

Healthy Fats and Oils

In a low-carb diet, healthy fats are essential for energy and satiety. Make sure to include these in your kitchen:

- **Oils:** Extra virgin olive oil, avocado oil, coconut oil, and ghee.

- **Butter:** Grass-fed butter is a great source of healthy fats.
- **Avocados:** A versatile fruit rich in healthy fats and fiber.

Sweeteners and Condiments

To keep your dishes flavorful without added sugars, consider these low-carb sweeteners and condiments:

- **Sweeteners:** Stevia, erythritol, monk fruit sweetener, and xylitol (use in moderation).
- **Condiments:** Mustard, mayonnaise (made with healthy oils), sugar-free ketchup, soy sauce (or tamari for gluten-free), hot sauce, and vinegar (apple cider, white, and balsamic).

Ingredient Substitutions

To make your favorite recipes low-carb friendly, here are some common ingredient substitutions:

- **Flour Substitutes:** Use almond flour or coconut flour instead of wheat flour in baking and cooking.
- **Pasta Substitutes:** Replace pasta with zucchini noodles (zoodles), spaghetti squash, or shirataki noodles.
- **Rice Substitutes:** Use cauliflower rice instead of white or brown rice.
- **Bread Substitutes:** Use lettuce wraps or make low-carb bread using almond flour or coconut flour recipes.
- **Sugar Substitutes:** Replace sugar with stevia, erythritol, or monk fruit sweetener in baking and beverages.

- **Potato Substitutes:** Use mashed cauliflower or turnips instead of mashed potatoes.

By stocking your kitchen with these essential low-carb foods, you'll be well-prepared to create a variety of delicious and nutritious meals that support your low-carb lifestyle. This approach makes it easier to stick to your diet and enjoy the many benefits of reduced carbohydrate intake.

CHAPTER 3

Meal Planning and Preparation

How to Plan Low-Carb Meals

Planning your meals ahead of time can help you stick to your low-carb diet, save time, and reduce stress during busy weeks. Here's how to effectively plan your low-carb meals:

→ **Set Your Goals**

- Determine your daily carb limit based on your personal goals (e.g., weight loss, blood sugar control).
- Decide on the number of meals and snacks you'll need for the week.

→ **Choose Your Recipes**

- Select a variety of recipes to keep your meals interesting. Include a mix of proteins, vegetables, and healthy fats.
- Consider different cooking methods to add variety (e.g., grilling, baking, slow-cooking).

→ **Create a Weekly Meal Plan**

- Plan your breakfasts, lunches, dinners, and snacks for each day.
- Ensure each meal includes a balance of proteins, fats, and low-carb vegetables.
- Write down your meal plan, using a template or a planner to keep organized.

→ **Prep in Advance**

- ◆ Prepare ingredients in bulk (e.g., chopping vegetables, cooking proteins) to save time during the week.
- ◆ Cook meals in larger batches and store portions in the refrigerator or freezer for easy access.

→ **Stay Flexible**

- ◆ Be prepared to adjust your meal plan if needed. Life can be unpredictable, and flexibility helps you stay on track.
- ◆ Have a few quick, go-to low-carb meals or snacks on hand for busy days.

Tips for Grocery Shopping

Smart grocery shopping is essential for maintaining a low-carb diet. Here are some tips to help you shop effectively:

1. **Make a Shopping List**
   a. Based on your meal plan, create a detailed shopping list of all the ingredients you'll need.
   b. Organize your list by categories (e.g., produce, dairy, meat) to make your shopping trip more efficient.

2. **Shop from the outer zone**
   a. Focus on the outer aisles of the grocery store, where fresh produce, meats, and dairy are typically located.
   b. Avoid the inner aisles, which are often filled with processed and high-carb foods.

3. **Read Labels**
   a. Check nutrition labels for hidden sugars and carbs. Look for foods with minimal ingredients and no added sugars.

    b. Pay attention to serving sizes to accurately calculate your carb intake.

4. **Stock Up on Staples**

    a. Keep your pantry stocked with low-carb staples like nuts, seeds, low-carb flours, and canned goods.

    b. Buy fresh produce, meats, and dairy regularly to ensure you have a steady supply of healthy ingredients.

5. **Buy in Bulk**

    a. Purchase bulk items like nuts, seeds, and meat to save money and reduce the frequency of shopping trips.

    b. Freeze bulk meats in portion sizes for easy thawing and cooking later.

6. **Avoid Temptations**

    a. Stick to your shopping list to avoid impulse buys.

    b. Avoid shopping when you're hungry to prevent purchasing high-carb, unhealthy foods.

7. **Look for Deals**

    a. Take advantage of sales and discounts on low-carb staples.

    b. Use coupons and store loyalty programs to save money on your grocery bills.

By planning your meals and shopping strategically, you can make your low-carb lifestyle more manageable and enjoyable. These steps will help you stay organized, save time, and ensure you always have nutritious, low-carb options available.

Batch Cooking and Meal Prep Strategies

Batch cooking and meal prep are excellent ways to ensure you have healthy, low-carb meals ready to go throughout the week. This approach saves time, reduces stress, and helps you stay on track with your diet. Here are some strategies for effective batch cooking and meal prep, along with tips for storing and freezing low-carb meals.

Batch Cooking Strategies

→ **Plan Your Menu**
  - Decide on a few recipes you want to make for the week. Aim for variety to keep your meals interesting.
  - Consider dishes that can be easily scaled up and stored, such as soups, stews, casseroles, and salads.

→ **Choose Versatile Ingredients**
  - Opt for ingredients that can be used in multiple dishes, such as grilled chicken, roasted vegetables, or cauliflower rice.
  - This approach allows you to mix and match components to create different meals.

→ **Cook in Bulk**
  - Prepare large batches of proteins (e.g., chicken breasts, ground beef), vegetables, and side dishes.
  - Use sheet pans, large pots, and slow cookers to cook multiple portions at once.

→ **Use Efficient Cooking Methods**
  - Utilize kitchen appliances like slow cookers, instant pots, and ovens to cook large quantities with minimal effort.

◆ Roasting vegetables and baking proteins simultaneously can save time and energy.

→ **Divide and Conquer**

◆ Divide your cooked food into individual portions for easy grab-and-go meals.

◆ Use portion control containers to ensure you have balanced meals ready to eat.

Meal Prep Strategies

❖ **Prep Ingredients Ahead of Time**

➢ Wash, chop, and portion out vegetables and fruits in advance.

➢ Marinate proteins and store them in the refrigerator until ready to cook.

❖ **Assemble Meals in Advance**

➢ Prepare complete meals and store them in the refrigerator for quick reheating.

➢ Layer salads in jars with dressing at the bottom and greens at the top to keep them fresh.

❖ **Label Everything**

➢ Clearly label containers with the contents and date of preparation to keep track of freshness.

➢ Use airtight containers to maintain the quality of your food.

❖ **Organize Your Fridge and Freezer**

➢ Keep your fridge and freezer organized to easily access prepped meals.

➢ Group similar items together and use clear containers to see what you have at a glance.

Storing and Freezing Low-Carb Meals

Proper storage is important in maintaining the quality and safety of your prepped meals. Below are some tips for storing and freezing low-carb meals:

1. **Refrigeration**
   a. Store cooked meals in airtight containers in the refrigerator for up to 4-5 days.
   b. Place the most perishable items at the front of the fridge to use them first.

2. **Freezing**
   a. Allow hot foods to cool before freezing to prevent condensation and ice crystals.
   b. Use freezer-safe containers or bags to store meals. Remove as much air as possible to prevent freezer burn.
   c. Label each container with the date and contents.

3. **Portion Control**
   a. Freeze meals in individual portions to make thawing and reheating more convenient.
   b. Consider using silicone muffin trays to freeze small portions of soups, sauces, and stews. Once frozen, transfer the portions to freezer bags.

4. **Thawing and Reheating**
   a. Thaw frozen meals in the refrigerator overnight for even defrosting.

    b. Reheat meals thoroughly, either in the microwave, on the stovetop, or in the oven, until they reach a safe internal temperature (165°F or 74°C).

5. **Storage Duration**

    a. Most cooked meals can be stored in the freezer for 2-3 months without significant loss of quality.

    b. Rotate your stock by placing newer items at the back and older items at the front to use them first.

By implementing these batch cooking and meal prep strategies, along with proper storage and freezing techniques, you can ensure you always have delicious and nutritious low-carb meals at your fingertips.

CHAPTER 4

Kitchen Essentials

Having the right tools and gadgets in your kitchen can make preparing low-carb meals easier, faster, and more enjoyable. Below is a comprehensive list of must-have kitchen essentials to support your low-carb lifestyle:

Basic Kitchen Tools

→ **Knives**

- ◆ **Chef's Knife:** A versatile knife for chopping, slicing, and dicing.
- ◆ **Paring Knife:** Ideal for peeling and intricate tasks.
- ◆ **Serrated Knife:** Perfect for cutting bread and tomatoes.

→ **Cutting Boards**

- ◆ **Wood or Bamboo Cutting Boards:** Gentle on knives and great for fruits, vegetables, and herbs.
- ◆ **Plastic Cutting Boards:** Easy to sanitize and ideal for meats and fish.

→ **Measuring Cups and Spoons**

- ◆ Essential for accurately measuring ingredients, especially when baking with low-carb flours.

→ **Mixing Bowls**

- ◆ A set of different sizes for mixing, marinating, and storing ingredients.

➔ **Colander/Strainer**

◆ Useful for washing vegetables, draining pasta substitutes like zucchini noodles, and rinsing canned beans.

➔ **Peeler**

◆ For peeling vegetables like carrots, cucumbers, and potatoes (or their low-carb substitutes).

Cooking Essentials

➔ **Pots and Pans**

◆ **Non-Stick Skillet:** Great for cooking eggs, meats, and stir-fries with minimal oil.

◆ **Saucepan:** For making sauces, soups, and boiling vegetables.

◆ **Stockpot:** Ideal for cooking large batches of soups, stews, and broth.

➔ **Baking Sheets**

◆ Versatile for roasting vegetables, baking low-carb treats, and making sheet pan dinners.

➔ **Cast Iron Skillet**

◆ Excellent for searing meats, baking, and one-pan meals.

➔ **Oven-Safe Baking Dishes**

◆ Useful for casseroles, baked dishes, and low-carb lasagnas.

➔ **Slow Cooker**

◆ Perfect for making stews, soups, and roasts with minimal effort.

➔ **Instant Pot**

◆ A multi-functional appliance that can pressure cook, slow cook, sauté, and more, making meal prep faster and easier.

➔ **Air Fryer**

◆ Great for making crispy, low-carb versions of traditionally fried foods with less oil.

Preparation Gadgets

→ **Food Processor**

◆ Essential for making cauliflower rice, chopping vegetables, and preparing low-carb doughs and batters.

→ **Blender**

◆ For smoothies, soups, sauces, and low-carb batters.

→ **Immersion Blender**

◆ Handy for blending soups and sauces directly in the pot.

→ **Spiralizer**

◆ Creates vegetable noodles from zucchini, carrots, and other vegetables, offering low-carb alternatives to pasta.

→ **Mandoline Slicer**

◆ For uniformly slicing vegetables, which is especially useful for dishes like zucchini lasagna and low-carb chips.

→ **Digital Kitchen Scale**

◆ Helps measure ingredients precisely, which is crucial for baking and portion control.

Storage Essentials

→ **Airtight Containers**

◆ Keep prepped ingredients and leftovers fresh. Glass containers are especially good for reheating food.

→ **Freezer Bags**

◆ For storing bulk-cooked meals and portioned ingredients in the freezer.

➜ **Mason Jars**

◆ Great for salads, dressings, and storing dry ingredients like nuts and seeds.

Additional Handy Tools

➜ **Grater/Zester**

◆ For grating cheese, zesting citrus, and shredding vegetables.

➜ **Tongs**

◆ Useful for flipping meats and vegetables, and serving salads.

➜ **Whisk**

◆ Essential for mixing batters, whipping cream, and combining ingredients.

➜ **Silicone Spatulas**

◆ Great for stirring, scraping bowls, and folding ingredients without scratching cookware.

➜ **Meat Thermometer**

◆ Ensures meats are cooked to the proper temperature, enhancing food safety and quality.

Having these essential kitchen tools and gadgets will streamline your meal preparation process and help you create a variety of delicious, low-carb dishes with ease. Investing in quality tools will not only make cooking more efficient but also more enjoyable, supporting your commitment to a low-carb lifestyle.

How to Use an Instant Pot

The Instant Pot is a versatile multi-cooker that combines several kitchen appliances into one, making it an essential tool for anyone following a low-carb diet. It can function as a pressure cooker, slow cooker, rice cooker, steamer, sauté pan, and more. Here's a guide to get you started with using your Instant Pot, along with some basics on slow cooking.

Getting Started with Your Instant Pot

1. **Read the Manual**
   - Before using your Instant Pot, familiarize yourself with the user manual to understand the various functions, safety features, and maintenance tips.

2. **Initial Setup**
   - Place the Instant Pot on a flat, stable surface near a power outlet.
   - Ensure the inner stainless steel pot is properly inserted.
   - Check that the silicone sealing ring is correctly fitted in the lid.

3. **Basic Controls and Functions**
   - **Pressure Cook:** The primary function for quick cooking. You can select High or Low pressure and set the cooking time.
   - **Sauté:** Use this function to brown meats, sauté vegetables, and simmer liquids before pressure cooking.
   - **Slow Cook:** Works like a traditional slow cooker with adjustable heat settings.
   - **Steam:** For steaming vegetables, fish, and more using the included steam rack.

- **Rice:** For perfectly cooked rice (or cauliflower rice) with the push of a button.
- **Yogurt:** For making homemade yogurt.

4. **Pressure Cooking Basics**
   - **Add Ingredients:** Place your ingredients into the inner pot. For pressure cooking, always add at least 1 cup of liquid (water, broth, etc.) to create the necessary steam.
   - **Seal the Lid:** Align the lid with the pot and turn it clockwise to lock it in place. Make sure the pressure release valve is set to the "Sealing" position.
   - **Select Pressure Cook Setting:** Press the "Pressure Cook" button and use the +/- buttons to adjust the cooking time. Select "High" or "Low" pressure if your model allows.
   - **Start Cooking:** The Instant Pot will take a few minutes to build pressure before the timer starts counting down.
   - **Release Pressure:** Once cooking is complete, you can release the pressure in two ways:
     - **Quick Release:** Turn the pressure release valve to the "Venting" position. Be cautious of the steam.
     - **Natural Release:** Let the pressure release naturally over time (10-20 minutes) before opening the lid.

5. **Cleaning and Maintenance**
   - Clean the inner pot, sealing ring, and lid after each use. The inner pot is usually dishwasher safe.
   - Wipe the outer housing with a damp cloth.
   - Check the sealing ring regularly for wear and replace it if necessary.

Slow Cooker Basics

The Instant Pot's slow cooker function can be a convenient way to prepare low-carb meals with minimal effort. Here are some basics for using the slow cooker feature:

1. **Setting Up**
   - Add your ingredients to the inner pot. There's no need for as much liquid as pressure cooking, but make sure the food is adequately covered or has enough moisture to prevent burning.

2. **Selecting the Slow Cook Function**
   - Place the lid on the Instant Pot and set the pressure release valve to "Venting" (this prevents pressure from building up).
   - Press the "Slow Cook" button. Use the "Adjust" button (if available) to set the cooking temperature to Low, Medium, or High.
   - Set the cooking time using the +/- buttons. Slow cooking times typically range from 4 to 10 hours, depending on the recipe and setting.

3. **Monitoring and Stirring**
   - Unlike pressure cooking, you can open the lid during slow cooking to stir or add ingredients. However, try to minimize this to maintain the cooking temperature.

4. **Tips for Best Results**
   - **Layering:** Place root vegetables at the bottom and meats on top, as the bottom layers cook faster.
   - **Herbs and Spices:** Add fresh herbs and delicate spices towards the end of the cooking time to retain their flavor.

- ○ **Liquid Reduction:** Slow cooking doesn't allow for much evaporation. If your dish is too liquidy, use the sauté function at the end to reduce the liquid.

By mastering the Instant Pot and its slow cooker function, you can effortlessly prepare a variety of delicious, low-carb meals, saving time and ensuring you always have nutritious options ready to enjoy.

Tips for Cooking Without Refined Carbs

Cooking without refined carbs can seem challenging at first, but with a few tips and substitutions, you can create delicious and nutritious meals that fit your low-carb lifestyle.Some strategies to help you get started are:

1. Understand Refined Carbs

- **What are Refined Carbs?** Refined carbs are processed foods that have had most of their fiber and nutrients removed. Common examples include white bread, pasta, pastries, and sugary snacks.
- **Why Avoid Them?** Refined carbs can cause rapid spikes in blood sugar levels, lead to weight gain, and contribute to various health issues.

2. Focus on Whole Foods

- **Vegetables:** Base your meals around non-starchy vegetables like leafy greens, broccoli, cauliflower, zucchini, and bell peppers.
- **Proteins:** Choose high-quality proteins such as chicken, beef, pork, fish, eggs, and plant-based options like tofu and tempeh.

- **Healthy Fats:** Incorporate healthy fats from avocados, nuts, seeds, olive oil, and coconut oil.

3. Use Low-Carb Substitutes

- **Flour Substitutes:** Replace wheat flour with almond flour, coconut flour, flaxseed meal, or a combination of low-carb flours.
- **Rice Substitutes:** Use cauliflower rice or broccoli rice instead of white or brown rice.
- **Pasta Substitutes:** Opt for zucchini noodles (zoodles), spaghetti squash, or shirataki noodles.
- **Bread Substitutes:** Use lettuce wraps, portobello mushroom caps, or make low-carb bread with almond or coconut flour.

4. Smart Snacking

- **Nuts and Seeds:** Almonds, walnuts, sunflower seeds, and chia seeds make excellent low-carb snacks.
- **Vegetables and Dip:** Pair raw vegetables with guacamole, hummus, or a low-carb yogurt dip.
- **Cheese:** Enjoy cheese slices or cheese sticks for a quick, satisfying snack.

5. Sweetener Alternatives

- **Natural Sweeteners:** Use stevia, erythritol, monk fruit sweetener, or xylitol instead of sugar. These sweeteners have minimal impact on blood sugar levels.
- **Fruits:** Incorporate small amounts of low-carb fruits like berries to add natural sweetness to your dishes.

6. Revamp Your Recipes

- **Baking:** Experiment with low-carb baking recipes using almond flour, coconut flour, and alternative sweeteners.
- **Breakfast:** Swap out traditional cereals and toast for low-carb options like eggs, avocado, and sautéed vegetables.
- **Lunch and Dinner:** Replace carb-heavy sides like potatoes and pasta with roasted vegetables, salads, and cauliflower mash.

7. Plan and Prepare

- **Meal Planning:** Plan your meals and snacks ahead of time to ensure you have low-carb options readily available.
- **Batch Cooking:** Prepare large batches of low-carb meals and store them in the fridge or freezer for quick and easy access.

8. Flavor Enhancements

- **Spices and Herbs:** Use a variety of spices and herbs to enhance the flavor of your dishes without adding carbs.
- **Condiments:** Opt for low-carb condiments like mustard, vinegar, hot sauce, and sugar-free ketchup.

9. Mindful Eating

- **Portion Control:** Be mindful of portion sizes, especially with nuts and low-carb treats, to avoid overconsumption.
- **Listen to Your Body:** Pay attention to hunger and fullness cues to avoid overeating.

10. Stay Hydrated

- **Drink Water:** Drinking plenty of water helps with digestion and can prevent cravings for carb-heavy snacks.
- **Low-Carb Beverages:** Enjoy beverages like herbal tea, black coffee, and sparkling water without added sugars.

CHAPTER 5

Breakfast Recipes

Classic Scrambled Eggs with Avocado

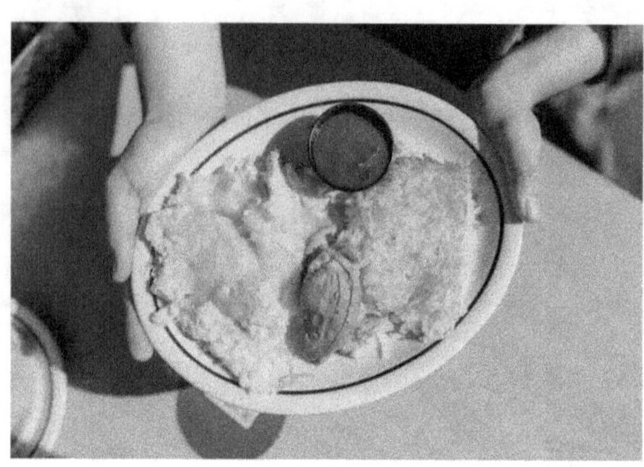

Ingredients:

- 4 large eggs
- 2 tablespoons heavy cream
- 1 tablespoon butter
- Salt and pepper to taste
- 1 ripe avocado, sliced
- 1 tablespoon chopped fresh chives (optional)

Instructions:

1. In a bowl, whisk together the eggs, heavy cream, salt, and pepper.
2. Heat the butter in a non-stick skillet over medium heat.
3. Pour the egg mixture into the skillet. Allow to sit for a few seconds, then gently stir with a spatula, pulling the eggs from the edges towards the center.
4. Continue to cook, stirring occasionally, until the eggs are softly set and slightly runny in places.
5. Remove from heat and let the residual heat finish cooking the eggs.
6. Serve with sliced avocado on the side. Sprinkle with chives if using.

Nutritional Information (per serving):

- Calories: 310
- Protein: 15g
- Fat: 28g
- Carbohydrates: 3g
- Fiber: 3g
- Net Carbs: 0g

Keto Pancakes with Almond Flour

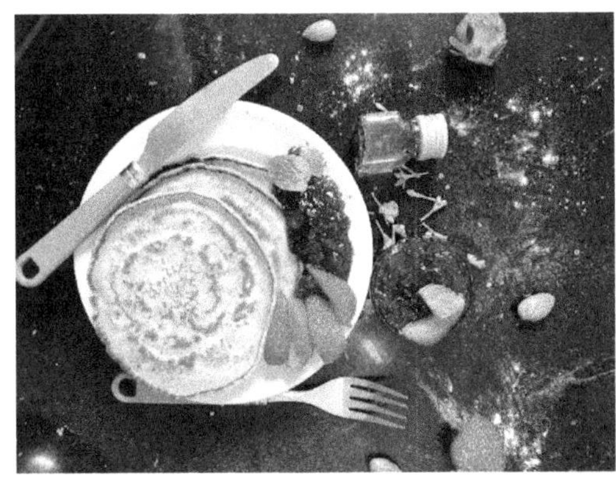

- 2 large eggs
- 1/4 cup unsweetened almond milk
- 1 tablespoon erythritol or preferred low-carb sweetener
- 1 teaspoon baking powder
- 1/4 teaspoon salt
- Butter or coconut oil for cooking

Ingredients:

- 1 cup almond flour

Instructions:

1. In a bowl, whisk together the almond flour, erythritol, baking powder, and salt.

2. In another bowl, beat the eggs and almond milk.

3. Combine the wet and dry ingredients, mixing until smooth.

4. Heat a non-stick skillet over medium heat and add a small amount of butter or coconut oil.

5. Pour batter onto the skillet to form small pancakes. Cook until bubbles form on the surface, then flip and cook until golden brown.

6. Serve with sugar-free syrup or berries.

Nutritional Information (per serving, makes 4 servings):

- Calories: 220
- Protein: 9g
- Fat: 18g
- Carbohydrates: 5g
- Fiber: 3g
- Net Carbs: 2g

Veggie-Packed Frittata

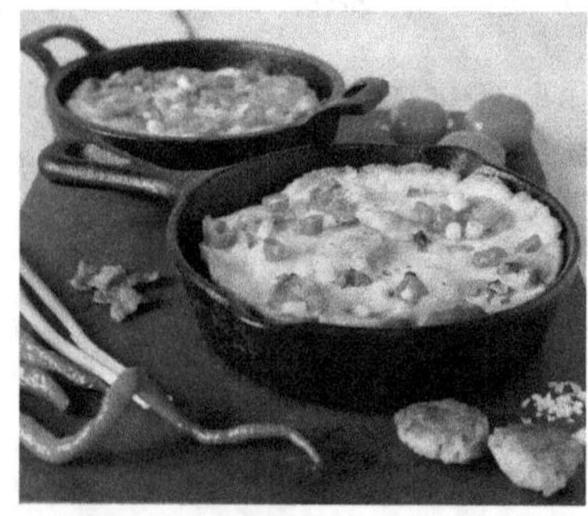

Ingredients:

- 6 large eggs
- 1/4 cup heavy cream
- 1 cup chopped spinach
- 1/2 cup diced bell pepper
- 1/2 cup sliced mushrooms
- 1/4 cup diced onion
- 1/2 cup shredded cheddar cheese
- 1 tablespoon olive oil
- Salt and pepper to taste

Instructions:

1. Preheat the oven to 350°F (175°C).

2. In a bowl, whisk together the eggs, heavy cream, salt, and pepper.

3. Heat olive oil in an oven-safe skillet over medium heat. Add the onion, bell pepper, and mushrooms, cooking until softened.

4. Add spinach and cook until wilted.

5. Pour the egg mixture over the vegetables and cook for a few minutes until the edges start to set.

6. Sprinkle the cheddar cheese on top and transfer the skillet to the oven.

7. Bake for 15-20 minutes, until the frittata is fully set and golden.

8. Let cool slightly before slicing and serving.

Nutritional Information (per serving, makes 4 servings):

- Calories: 220
- Protein: 14g
- Fat: 17g
- Carbohydrates: 5g
- Fiber: 2g
- Net Carbs: 3g

Chia Seed Pudding

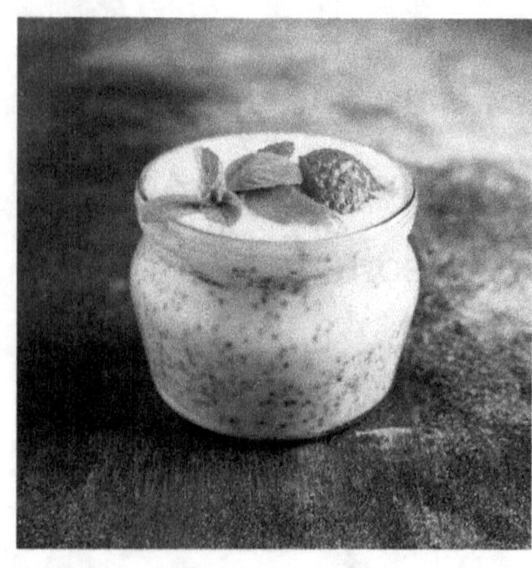

Ingredients:

- 1/4 cup chia seeds
- 1 cup unsweetened almond milk
- 1 tablespoon erythritol or preferred low-carb sweetener
- 1/2 teaspoon vanilla extract
- Fresh berries for topping (optional)

Instructions:

1. In a bowl or jar, mix chia seeds, almond milk, erythritol, and vanilla extract.
2. Stir well to ensure the chia seeds are evenly distributed.
3. Cover and refrigerate for at least 4 hours or overnight.
4. Stir before serving. Top with fresh berries if desired.

Nutritional Information (per serving, makes 2 servings):

- Calories: 150
- Protein: 5g
- Fat: 9g
- Carbohydrates: 12g
- Fiber: 10g
- Net Carbs: 2g

Instant Pot Egg Bites

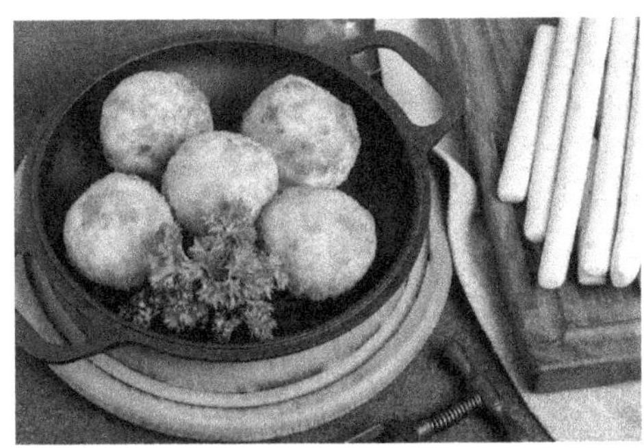

Ingredients:

- 6 large eggs
- 1/2 cup cottage cheese
- 1/2 cup shredded cheddar cheese
- 1/4 cup diced bacon or ham
- 1/4 cup chopped spinach
- Salt and pepper to taste

Instructions:

1. Blend the eggs and cottage cheese in a blender until smooth.
2. Stir in the cheddar cheese, bacon or ham, spinach, salt, and pepper.
3. Pour the mixture into silicone egg bite molds.
4. Add 1 cup of water to the Instant Pot and place the trivet inside.
5. Place the egg bite molds on the trivet, stacking if necessary.
6. Seal the lid and set the Instant Pot to Steam mode for 8 minutes.
7. Allow the pressure to release naturally for 10 minutes before quick releasing any remaining pressure.
8. Carefully remove the molds and let cool slightly before serving.

Nutritional Information (per serving, makes 6 servings):

- Calories: 140
- Protein: 10g
- Fat: 10g
- Carbohydrates: 2g
- Fiber: 0g
- Net Carbs: 2g

CHAPTER 6

Lunch Recipes

Zoodle (Zucchini Noodles) Salad with Pesto

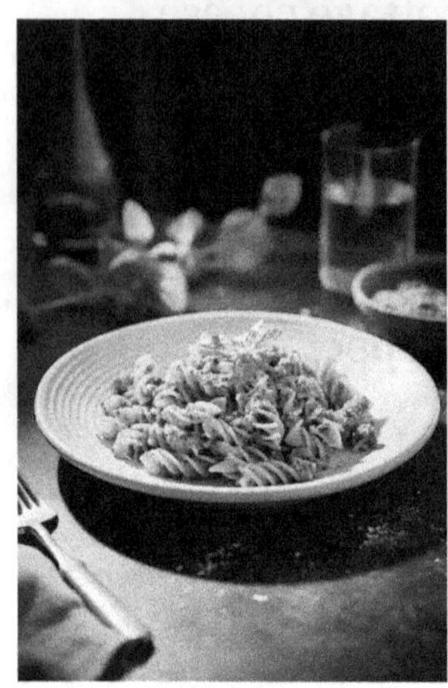

Ingredients:

- 2 medium zucchinis, spiralized into noodles
- 1 cup cherry tomatoes, halved
- 1/4 cup pine nuts, toasted
- 1/4 cup grated Parmesan cheese (optional)
- 1/2 cup fresh basil leaves
- 1/4 cup olive oil
- 1 clove garlic
- Salt and pepper to taste

Instructions:

1. In a food processor, combine basil, olive oil, garlic, and a pinch of salt and pepper. Blend until smooth to make the pesto.
2. In a large bowl, toss the zucchini noodles with the cherry tomatoes, pine nuts, and Parmesan cheese if using.
3. Add the pesto to the bowl and toss until the zoodles are evenly coated.
4. Serve immediately or chill for a refreshing cold salad.

Nutritional Information (per serving, makes 2 servings):

- Calories: 250
- Protein: 6g
- Fat: 22g
- Carbohydrates: 10g
- Fiber: 4g
- Net Carbs: 6g

<u>Cauliflower Rice Stir-Fry</u>

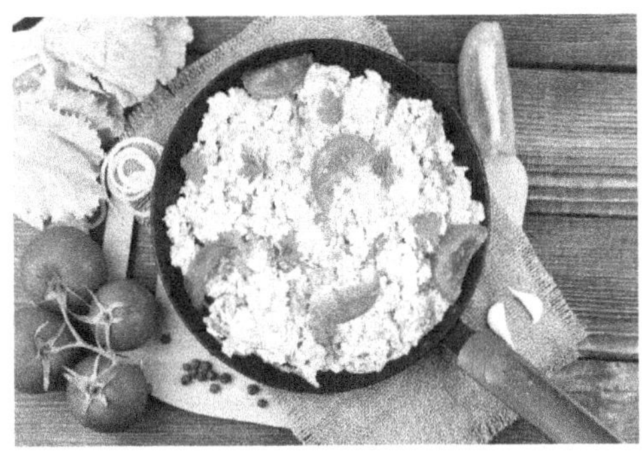

<u>Ingredients:</u>

- 1 medium head of cauliflower, grated into rice-sized pieces
- 1 cup mixed vegetables (e.g., bell peppers, peas, carrots, green beans), chopped
- 2 tablespoons soy sauce or tamari
- 1 tablespoon olive oil
- 2 large eggs, beaten
- 2 cloves garlic, minced
- 1/4 cup chopped green onions
- Salt and pepper to taste

<u>Instructions:</u>

1. Heat olive oil in a large skillet or wok over medium-high heat.
2. Add garlic and cook until fragrant, about 1 minute.
3. Add the mixed vegetables and stir-fry until tender, about 3-5 minutes.
4. Push the vegetables to one side of the skillet and pour the beaten eggs into the other side. Scramble the eggs until fully cooked.
5. Add the grated cauliflower and soy sauce to the skillet. Stir to combine everything.
6. Cook for another 3-5 minutes, until the cauliflower rice is tender but not mushy.
7. Season with salt and pepper, and stir in the green onions before serving.

Nutritional Information (per serving, makes 4 servings):

- Calories: 150
- Protein: 7g
- Fat: 8g
- Carbohydrates: 12g
- Fiber: 5g
- Net Carbs: 7g

Vegan Lentil Soup

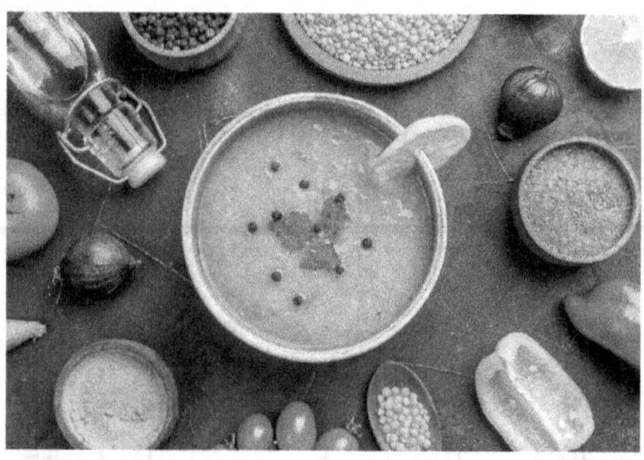

- 1 medium onion, diced
- 2 cloves garlic, minced
- 2 carrots, diced
- 2 celery stalks, diced
- 1 can (14.5 oz) diced tomatoes
- 4 cups vegetable broth
- 1 teaspoon cumin
- 1 teaspoon paprika
- 1/2 teaspoon turmeric
- Salt and pepper to taste
- 2 tablespoons olive oil

Ingredients:

- 1 cup dried lentils, rinsed and drained
- 2 cups fresh spinach, roughly chopped

Instructions:

1. Heat olive oil in a large pot over medium heat.

2. Add the onion, garlic, carrots, and celery. Sauté until vegetables are tender, about 5-7 minutes.

3. Stir in the cumin, paprika, turmeric, salt, and pepper. Cook for another 1-2 minutes.

4. Add the lentils, diced tomatoes, and vegetable broth to the pot. Bring to a boil.

5. Reduce heat and simmer for 30-40 minutes, until lentils are tender.

6. Stir in the fresh spinach and cook until wilted, about 2-3 minutes.

7. Adjust seasoning as needed and serve hot.

Nutritional Information (per serving, makes 4 servings):

- Calories: 210
- Protein: 10g
- Fat: 7g
- Carbohydrates: 30g
- Fiber: 12g
- Net Carbs: 18g

Cobb Salad with Low-Carb Dressing

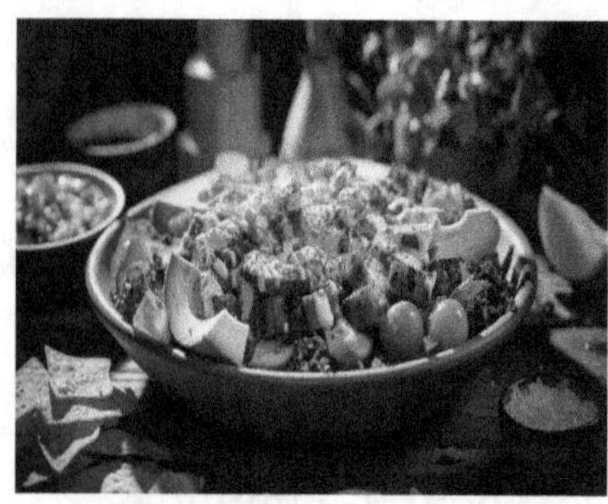

Ingredients:

- 4 cups mixed salad greens
- 1 large avocado, diced
- 2 hard-boiled eggs, chopped
- 1 cup cooked chicken breast, diced
- 1/2 cup cherry tomatoes, halved
- 1/4 cup blue cheese, crumbled
- 4 slices cooked bacon, crumbled

Low-Carb Dressing:

- 1/4 cup olive oil
- 2 tablespoons apple cider vinegar
- 1 tablespoon Dijon mustard
- 1 clove garlic, minced
- Salt and pepper to taste

Instructions:

1. In a large bowl, arrange the salad greens as the base.
2. Top with avocado, hard-boiled eggs, chicken breast, cherry tomatoes, blue cheese, and bacon.
3. In a small bowl, whisk together the olive oil, apple cider vinegar, Dijon mustard, garlic, salt, and pepper to make the dressing.
4. Drizzle the dressing over the salad just before serving and toss to combine.

Nutritional Information (per serving, makes 2 servings):

- Calories: 450
- Protein: 30g
- Fat: 35g
- Carbohydrates: 8g
- Fiber: 5g
- Net Carbs: 3g

Slow Cooker Vegetable Stew

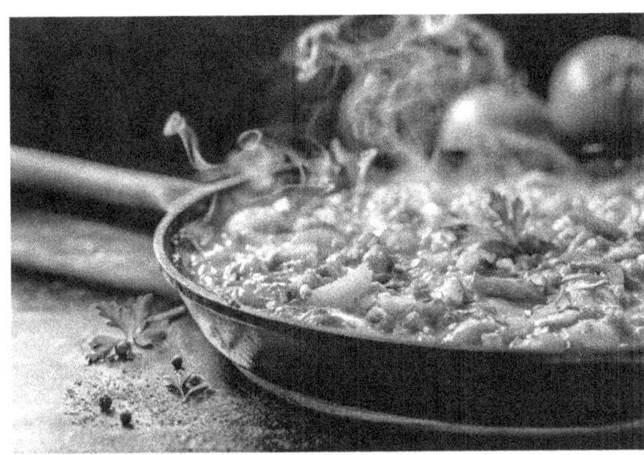

Ingredients:

- 2 cups diced tomatoes
- 1 medium zucchini, chopped
- 1 medium bell pepper, chopped
- 1 medium onion, chopped
- 2 cloves garlic, minced
- 2 cups vegetable broth
- 1 cup chopped carrots
- 1 cup chopped green beans
- 1 teaspoon dried thyme
- 1 teaspoon dried basil
- 1/2 teaspoon salt
- 1/4 teaspoon pepper

Instructions:

1. Add all the ingredients to a slow cooker and stir to combine.
2. Cover and cook on low for 6-8 hours or on high for 3-4 hours, until vegetables are tender.
3. Adjust seasoning if needed before serving.

Nutritional Information (per serving, makes 4 servings):

- Calories: 120
- Protein: 3g
- Fat: 2g
- Carbohydrates: 22g
- Fiber: 7g
- Net Carbs: 15g

CHAPTER 7

Dinner Recipes

Baked Salmon with Asparagus

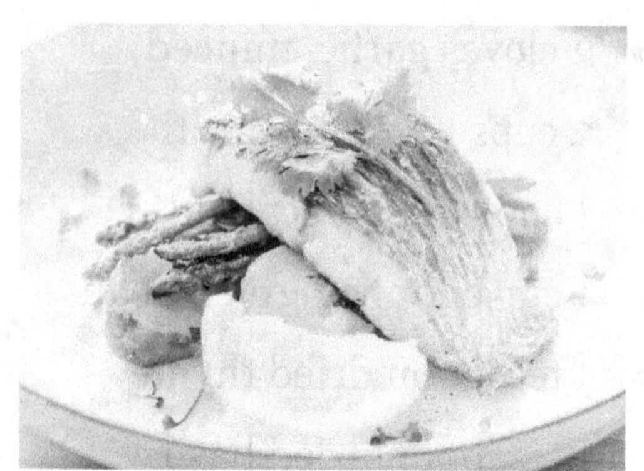

Ingredients:

- 4 salmon fillets (about 6 ounces each)
- 1 bunch asparagus, trimmed
- 2 tablespoons olive oil
- 2 cloves garlic, minced
- 1 lemon, sliced
- Salt and pepper to taste
- Fresh dill or parsley for garnish (optional)

Instructions:

1. Preheat the oven to 400°F (200°C).
2. Line a baking sheet with parchment paper or foil.
3. Arrange the salmon fillets and asparagus on the baking sheet.
4. Drizzle with olive oil and sprinkle with minced garlic, salt, and pepper.
5. Place lemon slices on top of the salmon fillets.
6. Bake for 15-20 minutes, until the salmon is cooked through and the asparagus is tender.
7. Garnish with fresh dill or parsley before serving if desired.

Nutritional Information (per serving, makes 4 servings):

- Calories: 350
- Protein: 30g
- Fat: 22g
- Carbohydrates: 6g
- Fiber: 3g
- Net Carbs: 3g

<u>**Stuffed Bell Peppers**</u>

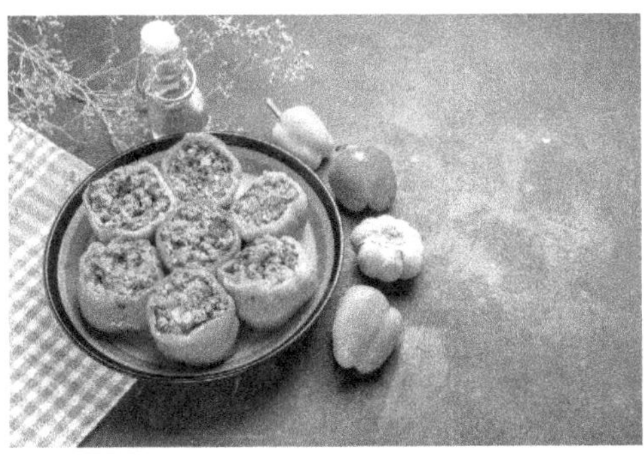

Ingredients:

- 4 large bell peppers, tops cut off and seeds removed
- 1 pound ground beef or turkey
- 1 small onion, diced
- 2 cloves garlic, minced
- 1 cup cauliflower rice
- 1 cup diced tomatoes
- 1 cup shredded cheese (cheddar or mozzarella)
- 1 tablespoon olive oil
- 1 teaspoon dried oregano
- 1 teaspoon dried basil
- Salt and pepper to taste

Instructions:

1. Preheat the oven to 375°F (190°C).
2. In a large skillet, heat olive oil over medium heat. Add the onion and garlic, cooking until soft.
3. Add the ground beef or turkey and cook until browned. Drain any excess fat.
4. Stir in the cauliflower rice, diced tomatoes, oregano, basil, salt, and pepper. Cook for another 5-7 minutes.
5. Remove from heat and stir in half of the shredded cheese.
6. Stuff each bell pepper with the meat mixture and place in a baking dish.
7. Top with the remaining cheese and cover with foil.
8. Bake for 30 minutes, then remove the foil and bake for an additional 10 minutes until the peppers are tender and the cheese is bubbly.

<u>Nutritional Information (per serving, makes 4 servings):</u>

- Calories: 320
- Protein: 28g
- Fat: 18g
- Carbohydrates: 10g
- Fiber: 3g
- Net Carbs: 7g

<u>Eggplant Lasagna</u>

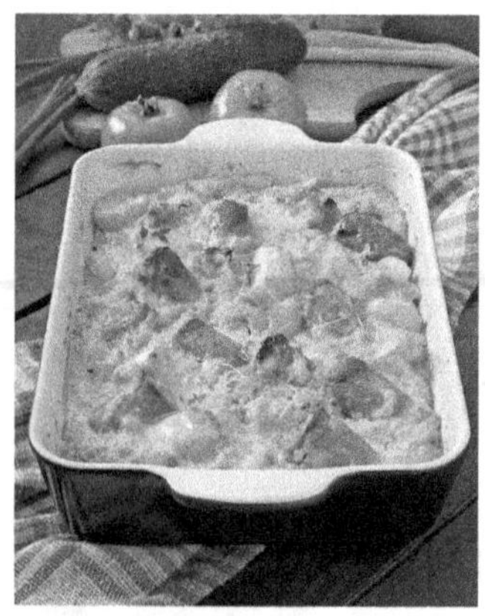

- 1 small onion, diced
- 2 cloves garlic, minced
- 1 can (14.5 oz) diced tomatoes
- 1 cup ricotta cheese
- 2 cups shredded mozzarella cheese
- 1/2 cup grated Parmesan cheese
- 1 egg, beaten
- 2 tablespoons olive oil
- 1 teaspoon dried oregano
- 1 teaspoon dried basil
- Salt and pepper to taste

<u>Ingredients:</u>

- 2 large eggplants, sliced lengthwise into 1/4-inch thick slices
- 1 pound ground beef or turkey

<u>Instructions:</u>

1. Preheat the oven to 375°F (190°C).

2. Sprinkle the eggplant slices with salt and let sit for 15 minutes to draw out moisture. Pat dry with paper towels.

3. In a large skillet, heat olive oil over medium heat. Add the onion and garlic, cooking until soft.

4. Add the ground beef or turkey and cook until browned. Drain any excess fat.

5. Stir in the diced tomatoes, oregano, basil, salt, and pepper. Simmer for 10 minutes.

6. In a bowl, combine the ricotta cheese, Parmesan cheese, and beaten egg.

7. In a baking dish, layer half of the eggplant slices, followed by half of the meat mixture, then half of the ricotta mixture, and half of the mozzarella cheese. Repeat the layers.

8. Cover with foil and bake for 30 minutes. Remove the foil and bake for an additional 10-15 minutes until the cheese is bubbly and golden.

Nutritional Information (per serving, makes 6 servings):

- Calories: 340
- Protein: 28g
- Fat: 22g
- Carbohydrates: 12g
- Fiber: 5g
- Net Carbs: 7g

Vegan Cauliflower Curry

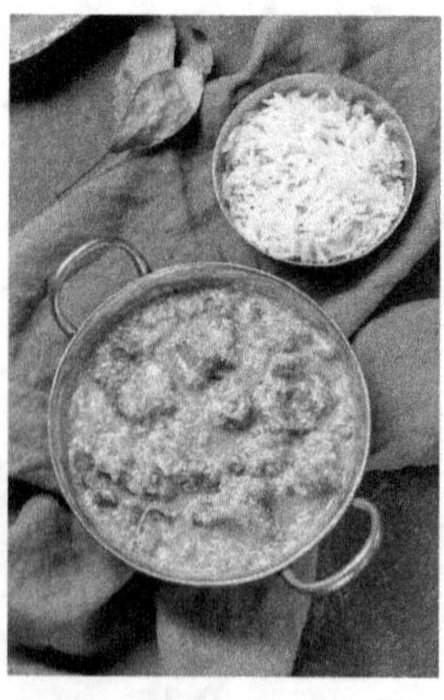

- 1 can (14 oz) coconut milk
- 1 medium onion, diced
- 2 cloves garlic, minced
- 1 tablespoon ginger, minced
- 2 tablespoons curry powder
- 1 teaspoon ground cumin
- 1 teaspoon ground turmeric
- 1/2 teaspoon cayenne pepper (optional)
- 2 tablespoons coconut oil
- Salt and pepper to taste
- Fresh cilantro for garnish (optional)

Ingredients:

- 1 large head of cauliflower, cut into florets
- 1 can (14.5 oz) diced tomatoes

Instructions:

1. In a large pot, heat the coconut oil over medium heat. Add the onion, garlic, and ginger, cooking until soft.
2. Stir in the curry powder, cumin, turmeric, and cayenne pepper. Cook for 1-2 minutes until fragrant.
3. Add the diced tomatoes and coconut milk, stirring to combine.
4. Add the cauliflower florets, salt, and pepper. Bring to a simmer and cook for 20-25 minutes until the cauliflower is tender.
5. Adjust seasoning if needed. Garnish with fresh cilantro before serving.

Nutritional Information (per serving, makes 4 servings):

- Calories: 220
- Protein: 5g
- Fat: 18g
- Carbohydrates: 14g
- Fiber: 5g
- Net Carbs: 9g

Instant Pot Chicken Thighs with Mushrooms

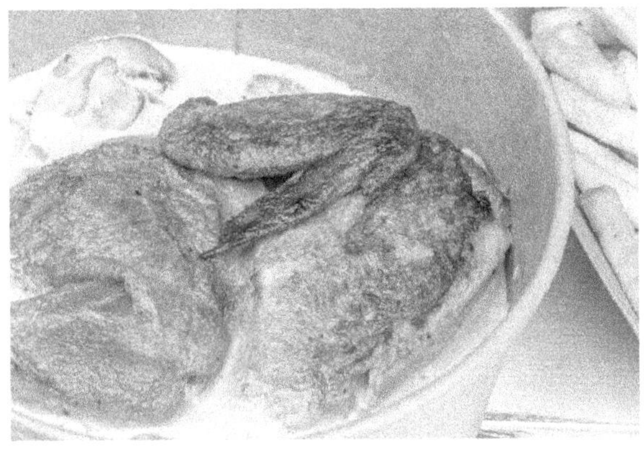

- 2 cups sliced mushrooms
- 1 medium onion, diced
- 3 cloves garlic, minced
- 1 cup chicken broth
- 1/2 cup heavy cream
- 2 tablespoons olive oil
- 1 teaspoon dried thyme
- 1 teaspoon dried rosemary
- Salt and pepper to taste
- Fresh parsley for garnish (optional)

Ingredients:

- 6 bone-in, skin-on chicken thighs

Instructions:

1. Season the chicken thighs with salt and pepper.

2. Set the Instant Pot to sauté mode and heat the olive oil. Add the chicken thighs, skin side down, and brown for 4-5 minutes. Flip and brown the other side for another 3-4 minutes. Remove and set aside.

3. Add the onion and garlic to the Instant Pot and sauté until softened.

4. Stir in the mushrooms, thyme, and rosemary, cooking for another 2-3 minutes.

5. Pour in the chicken broth and use a wooden spoon to scrape up any browned bits from the bottom.

6. Return the chicken thighs to the Instant Pot. Secure the lid and set the pressure release valve to sealing.

7. Cook on high pressure for 10 minutes. Allow the pressure to release naturally for 10 minutes, then quick release any remaining pressure.

8. Remove the chicken thighs and set the Instant Pot to sauté mode. Stir in the heavy cream and cook for a few minutes until the sauce thickens slightly.

9. Serve the chicken thighs with the mushroom sauce. Garnish with fresh parsley if desired.

Nutritional Information (per serving, makes 4 servings):

- Calories: 450
- Protein: 28g
- Fat: 34g
- Carbohydrates: 6g
- Fiber: 1g
- Net Carbs: 5g

CHAPTER 8

Snacks and Sides Recipes

<u>Avocado Deviled Eggs</u>

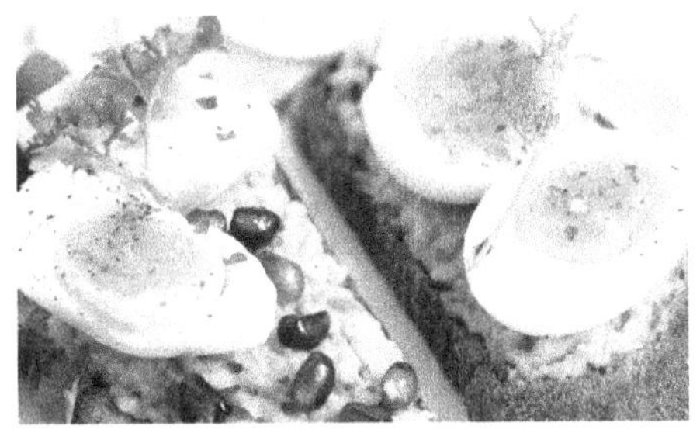

Ingredients:

- 6 large eggs
- 1 ripe avocado, peeled and pitted
- 1 tablespoon lime juice
- 2 tablespoons mayonnaise
- 1 teaspoon Dijon mustard
- Salt and pepper to taste
- Paprika for garnish (optional)
- Fresh cilantro for garnish (optional)

Instructions:

1. Place the eggs in a saucepan and cover with water. Bring to a boil, then remove from heat and let sit for 12 minutes. Transfer the eggs to an ice bath to cool.

2. Peel the eggs and cut them in half lengthwise. Remove the yolks and place them in a bowl.

3. Add the avocado, lime juice, mayonnaise, Dijon mustard, salt, and pepper to the bowl with the yolks. Mash and mix until smooth.

4. Spoon the avocado mixture back into the egg whites.

5. Garnish with paprika and fresh cilantro if desired. Serve immediately or chill until ready to serve.

Nutritional Information (per serving, makes 6 servings):

- Calories: 120
- Protein: 6g
- Fat: 10g
- Carbohydrates: 2g
- Fiber: 1g
- Net Carbs: 1g

Spicy Roasted Chickpeas

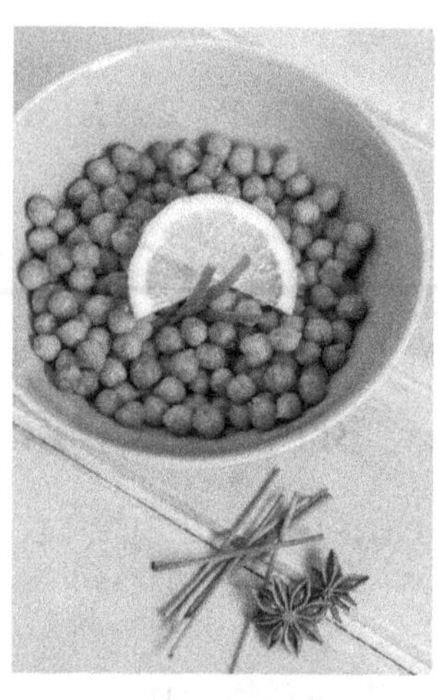

Ingredients:

- 1 can (15 oz) chickpeas, rinsed and drained
- 2 tablespoons olive oil
- 1 teaspoon chili powder
- 1/2 teaspoon cumin
- 1/2 teaspoon paprika
- 1/4 teaspoon cayenne pepper (optional)
- Salt and pepper to taste

Instructions:

1. Preheat the oven to 400°F (200°C).
2. Pat the chickpeas dry with paper towels.
3. In a bowl, toss the chickpeas with olive oil, chili powder, cumin, paprika, cayenne pepper, salt, and pepper.
4. Spread the chickpeas in a single layer on a baking sheet.

5. Roast for 20-30 minutes, shaking the pan occasionally, until the chickpeas are crispy.
6. Let cool slightly before serving.

Nutritional Information (per serving, makes 4 servings):

- Calories: 120
- Protein: 5g
- Fat: 7g
- Carbohydrates: 12g
- Fiber: 4g
- Net Carbs: 8g

Kale Chips

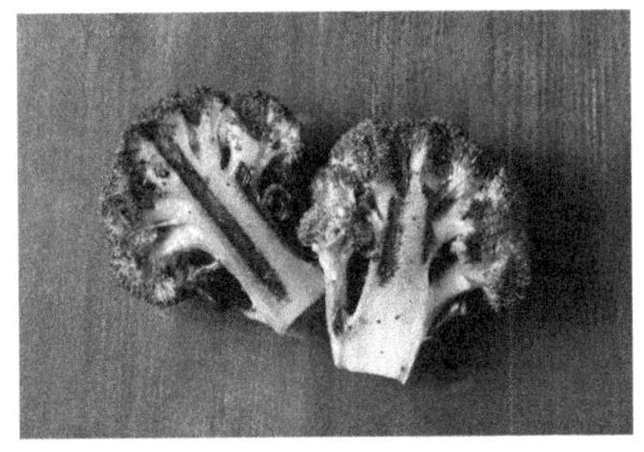

Ingredients:

- 1 bunch kale, washed and thoroughly dried
- 1 tablespoon olive oil
- 1/2 teaspoon sea salt
- 1/4 teaspoon garlic powder (optional)

Instructions:

1. Preheat the oven to 300°F (150°C).
2. Remove the kale leaves from the stems and tear into bite-sized pieces.

3. In a large bowl, toss the kale with olive oil, sea salt, and garlic powder if using.

4. Spread the kale in a single layer on a baking sheet.

5. Bake for 20-25 minutes, until the edges are brown but not burnt, and the kale is crispy.

6. Let cool before serving.

Nutritional Information (per serving, makes 4 servings):

- Calories: 50
- Protein: 2g
- Fat: 3g
- Carbohydrates: 5g
- Fiber: 2g
- Net Carbs: 3g

Guacamole with Cucumber Slices

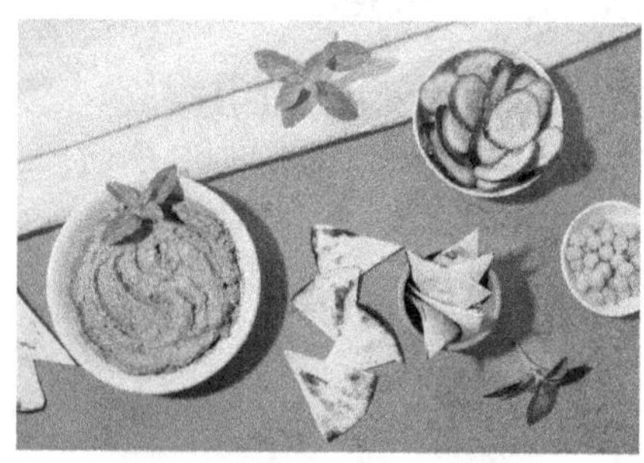

Ingredients:

- 2 ripe avocados, peeled and pitted
- 1 tablespoon lime juice
- 1 small tomato, diced
- 1/4 cup red onion, finely chopped
- 1 clove garlic, minced
- 1 tablespoon fresh cilantro, chopped
- Salt and pepper to taste
- 1 large cucumber, sliced

Instructions:

1. In a bowl, mash the avocados with lime juice until smooth.
2. Stir in the diced tomato, red onion, garlic, cilantro, salt, and pepper.
3. Serve the guacamole with cucumber slices for dipping.

Nutritional Information (per serving, makes 4 servings):

- Calories: 160
- Protein: 2g
- Fat: 14g
- Carbohydrates: 9g
- Fiber: 5g
- Net Carbs: 4g

Cauliflower Mash

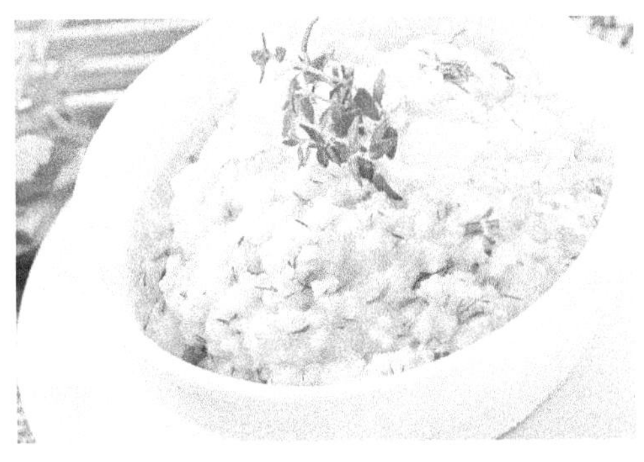

- 1 large head cauliflower, cut into florets
- 2 tablespoons butter
- 1/4 cup heavy cream
- 1 clove garlic, minced

Ingredients:

- Salt and pepper to taste
- Fresh chives for garnish (optional)

Instructions:

1. Bring a large pot of salted water to a boil. Add the cauliflower florets and cook until tender, about 10-12 minutes.
2. Drain the cauliflower and return it to the pot.
3. Add the butter, heavy cream, garlic, salt, and pepper. Use an immersion blender or a potato masher to mash the cauliflower until smooth.
4. Adjust seasoning to taste.
5. Garnish with fresh chives if desired and serve hot.

Nutritional Information (per serving, makes 4 servings):

- Calories: 120
- Protein: 3g
- Fat: 10g
- Carbohydrates: 7g
- Fiber: 3g
- Net Carbs: 4g

CHAPTER 9

Desserts Recipes

Chocolate Avocado Mousse

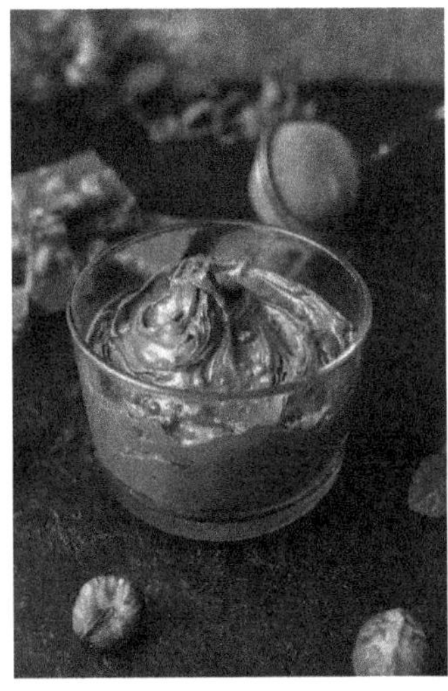

Ingredients:

- 2 ripe avocados, peeled and pitted
- 1/4 cup unsweetened cocoa powder
- 1/4 cup maple syrup or a low-carb sweetener of choice
- 1/4 cup almond milk or coconut milk
- 1 teaspoon vanilla extract
- A pinch of sal

Instructions:

1. In a food processor, combine the avocados, cocoa powder, maple syrup, almond milk, vanilla extract, and salt.
2. Blend until smooth and creamy.
3. Chill in the refrigerator for at least 30 minutes before serving.
4. Garnish with fresh berries or a sprinkle of cocoa powder if desired.

Nutritional Information (per serving, makes 4 servings):

- Calories: 180
- Protein: 2g
- Fat: 15g
- Carbohydrates: 15g
- Fiber: 7g
- Net Carbs: 8g

Coconut Flour Brownies

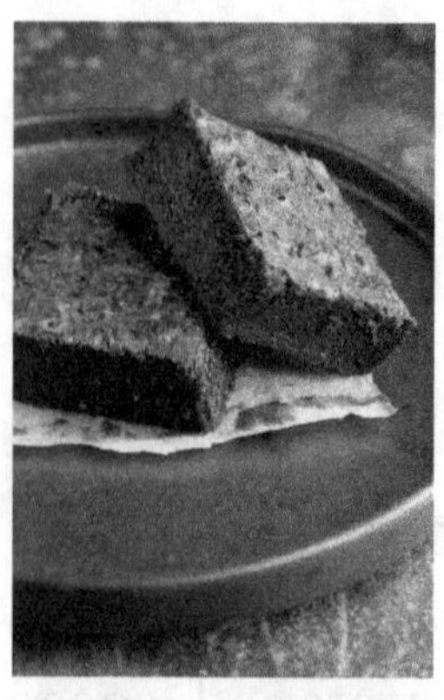

Ingredients:

- 1/2 cup coconut flour
- 1/2 cup unsweetened cocoa powder
- 1/4 teaspoon baking powder
- 1/4 teaspoon salt
- 4 large eggs
- 1/2 cup coconut oil or butter, melted
- 1/2 cup low-carb sweetener (e.g., erythritol or stevia)
- 1 teaspoon vanilla extract

Instructions:

1. Preheat the oven to 350°F (175°C). Grease an 8x8-inch baking pan or line with parchment paper.
2. In a bowl, whisk together the coconut flour, cocoa powder, baking powder, and salt.
3. In another bowl, beat the eggs, then add the melted coconut oil, sweetener, and vanilla extract.
4. Combine the wet and dry ingredients and mix until smooth.
5. Pour the batter into the prepared pan and spread evenly.
6. Bake for 20-25 minutes, or until a toothpick inserted in the center comes out clean.
7. Let cool before cutting into squares.

Nutritional Information (per serving, makes 9 servings):

- Calories: 180
- Protein: 4g
- Fat: 15g
- Carbohydrates: 13g
- Fiber: 6g
- Net Carbs: 7g

Berry Parfait with Whipped Cream

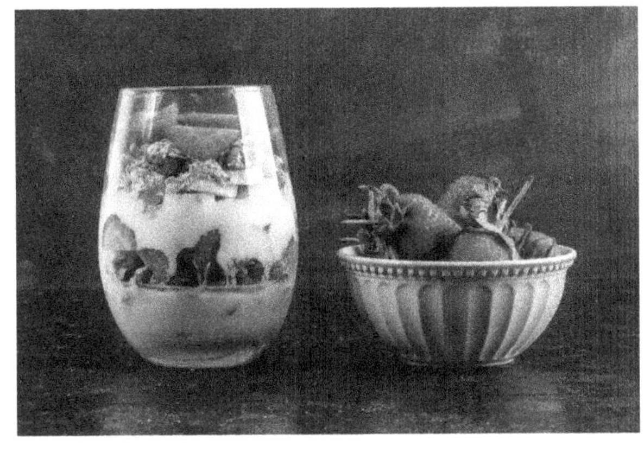

Ingredients:

- 1 cup mixed berries (strawberries, blueberries, raspberries)
- 1 cup heavy cream
- 2 tablespoons powdered erythritol or another low-carb sweetener
- 1/2 teaspoon vanilla extract

Instructions:

1. In a mixing bowl, whip the heavy cream with a hand mixer or stand mixer until soft peaks form.

2. Add the sweetener and vanilla extract and continue to whip until stiff peaks form.
3. In serving glasses, layer the mixed berries with the whipped cream.
4. Repeat the layers until the glasses are full.
5. Serve immediately or chill in the refrigerator until ready.

Nutritional Information (per serving, makes 4 servings):

- Calories: 150
- Protein: 2g
- Fat: 15g
- Carbohydrates: 10g
- Fiber: 4g
- Net Carbs: 6g

Vegan Fat Bombs

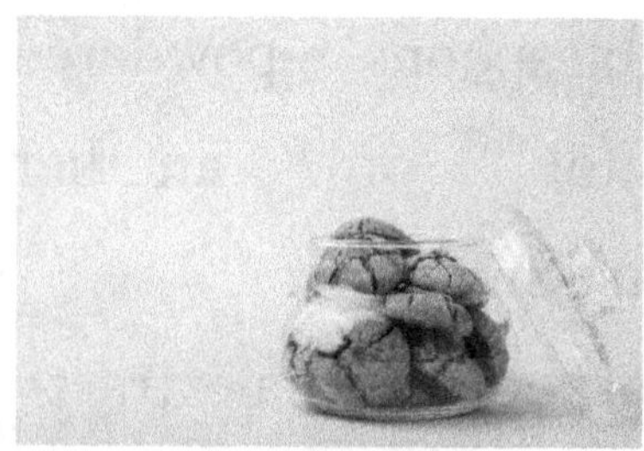

Ingredients:

- 1/2 cup coconut oil, melted
- 1/4 cup almond butter or peanut butter
- 1/4 cup unsweetened cocoa powder
- 2 tablespoons powdered erythritol or another low-carb sweetener
- 1/2 teaspoon vanilla extract

Instructions:

1. In a bowl, combine the melted coconut oil, almond butter, cocoa powder, sweetener, and vanilla extract.
2. Mix until well combined and smooth.
3. Pour the mixture into silicone molds or mini muffin tins.
4. Refrigerate for at least 30 minutes until solid.
5. Pop out of molds and store in the refrigerator.

Nutritional Information (per serving, makes 12 servings):

- Calories: 120
- Protein: 3g
- Fat: 10g
- Carbohydrates: 8g
- Fiber: 4g
- Net Carbs: 4g

Instant Pot Cheesecake

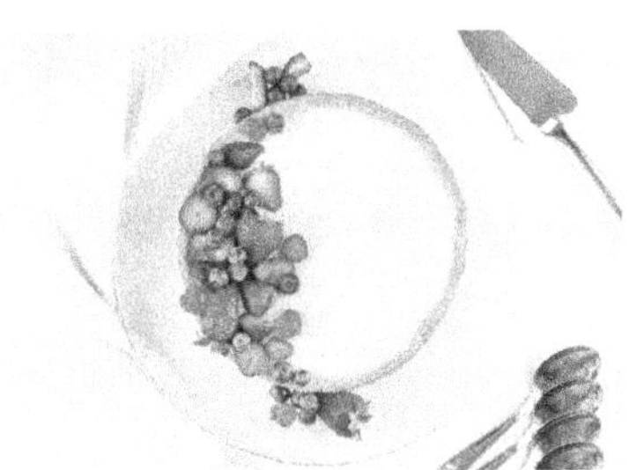

Ingredients:

- 1 1/2 cups almond flour
- 1/4 cup melted butter
- 2 cups cream cheese, softened
- 1/2 cup sour cream
- 1/2 cup low-carb sweetener (e.g., erythritol or stevia)
- 3 large eggs
- 1 teaspoon vanilla extract
- 1/2 teaspoon lemon zest (optional)

Instructions:

1. In a bowl, mix the almond flour and melted butter until well combined. Press the mixture into the bottom of a springform pan.
2. In a large bowl, beat the cream cheese until smooth. Add the sour cream, sweetener, eggs, vanilla extract, and lemon zest if using. Mix until smooth and well combined.
3. Pour the cream cheese mixture over the crust in the springform pan.
4. Cover the pan with foil to prevent condensation.
5. Pour 1 cup of water into the Instant Pot and place a trivet inside.
6. Set the springform pan on the trivet and close the Instant Pot lid. Set to high pressure for 35 minutes.
7. Allow the pressure to release naturally. Remove the cheesecake and let it cool to room temperature, then refrigerate for at least 4 hours before serving.

Nutritional Information (per serving, makes 8 servings):

- Calories: 290
- Protein: 7g
- Fat: 24g
- Carbohydrates: 7g
- Fiber: 1g
- Net Carbs: 6g

CHAPTER 10

Vegan and Vegetarian Options

<u>High-Protein Vegan Chili</u>

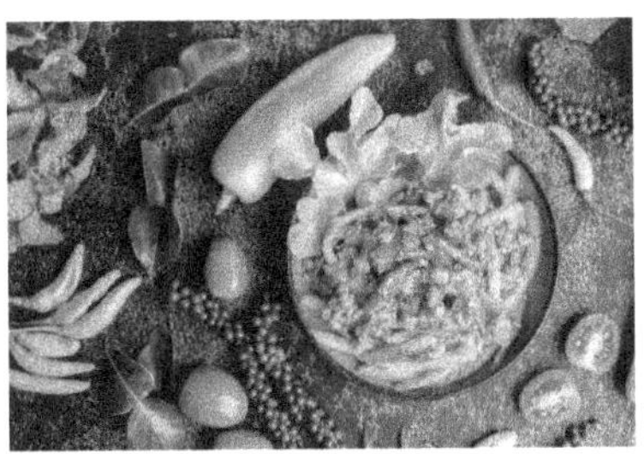

Ingredients:

- 1 tablespoon olive oil
- 1 large onion, diced
- 2 cloves garlic, minced
- 1 bell pepper, diced
- 2 cups cooked black beans
- 1 cup cooked quinoa
- 1 can (14.5 oz) diced tomatoes
- 1 cup vegetable broth
- 1 can (15 oz) kidney beans, rinsed and drained
- 1 cup corn kernels (optional)
- 2 tablespoons chili powder
- 1 teaspoon ground cumin
- 1 teaspoon smoked paprika
- Salt and pepper to taste
- Fresh cilantro for garnish (optional)

Instructions:

1. Heat the olive oil in a large pot over medium heat. Add the onion, garlic, and bell pepper, cooking until softened.
2. Stir in the chili powder, cumin, and smoked paprika. Cook for 1-2 minutes.
3. Add the diced tomatoes, vegetable broth, black beans, quinoa, kidney beans, and corn if using.

4. Bring to a boil, then reduce heat and simmer for 20-25 minutes, until the chili is thickened and flavors are blended.

5. Adjust seasoning with salt and pepper. Garnish with fresh cilantro if desired before serving.

Nutritional Information (per serving, makes 6 servings):

- Calories: 220
- Protein: 12g
- Fat: 4g
- Carbohydrates: 36g
- Fiber: 8g
- Net Carbs: 28g

Stuffed Portobello Mushrooms

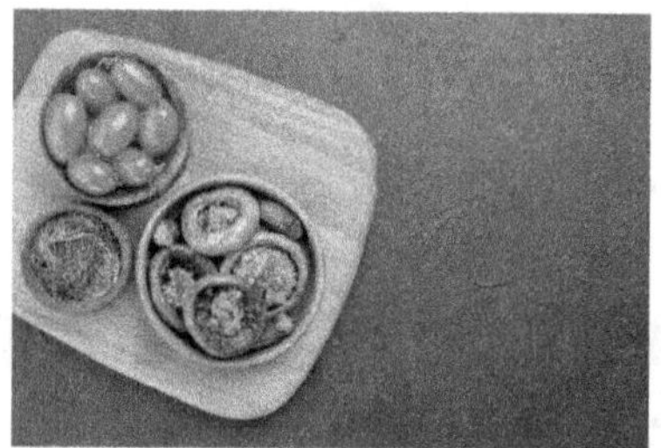

Ingredients:

- 4 large portobello mushrooms, stems removed
- 1 cup cooked quinoa
- 1/2 cup sun-dried tomatoes, chopped
- 1/4 cup pine nuts, toasted
- 1/2 cup spinach, chopped
- 2 cloves garlic, minced
- 1 tablespoon olive oil
- Salt and pepper to taste
- 1/4 cup vegan Parmesan cheese (optional)

Instructions:

1. Preheat the oven to 375°F (190°C).
2. In a skillet, heat olive oil over medium heat. Add garlic and cook until fragrant.
3. Stir in the sun-dried tomatoes, spinach, and cooked quinoa. Cook until the spinach is wilted.
4. Remove from heat and mix in the pine nuts. Season with salt and pepper.
5. Place the portobello mushrooms on a baking sheet and fill each with the quinoa mixture.
6. Top with vegan Parmesan cheese if desired.
7. Bake for 20-25 minutes, until the mushrooms are tender and the topping is golden.

Nutritional Information (per serving, makes 4 servings):

- Calories: 180
- Protein: 7g
- Fat: 10g
- Carbohydrates: 18g
- Fiber: 4g
- Net Carbs: 14g

Tofu Stir-Fry with Broccoli

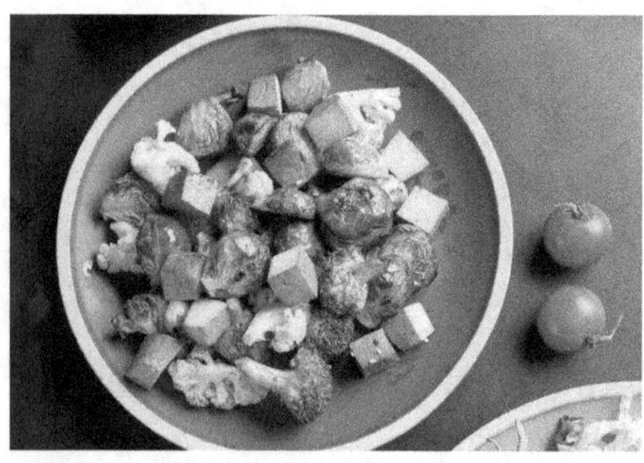

Ingredients:

- 1 block (14 oz) firm tofu, pressed and cubed
- 2 tablespoons soy sauce or tamari
- 1 tablespoon hoisin sauce (check for low-carb version)
- 2 tablespoons sesame oil
- 2 cups broccoli florets
- 1 red bell pepper, sliced
- 1/2 cup snap peas
- 2 cloves garlic, minced
- 1 teaspoon grated ginger
- 1 tablespoon sesame seeds (optional)

Instructions:

1. In a large skillet or wok, heat sesame oil over medium-high heat. Add tofu and cook until golden brown on all sides. Remove from the skillet and set aside.
2. In the same skillet, add garlic and ginger, cooking until fragrant.
3. Add the broccoli, bell pepper, and snap peas. Stir-fry for 4-5 minutes, until the vegetables are tender-crisp.
4. Return the tofu to the skillet. Add soy sauce and hoisin sauce, stirring to coat evenly.
5. Cook for an additional 2 minutes, until everything is heated through.
6. Garnish with sesame seeds if desired before serving.

Nutritional Information (per serving, makes 4 servings):

- Calories: 200
- Protein: 15g
- Fat: 14g
- Carbohydrates: 12g
- Fiber: 5g
- Net Carbs: 7g

Spaghetti Squash with Marinara

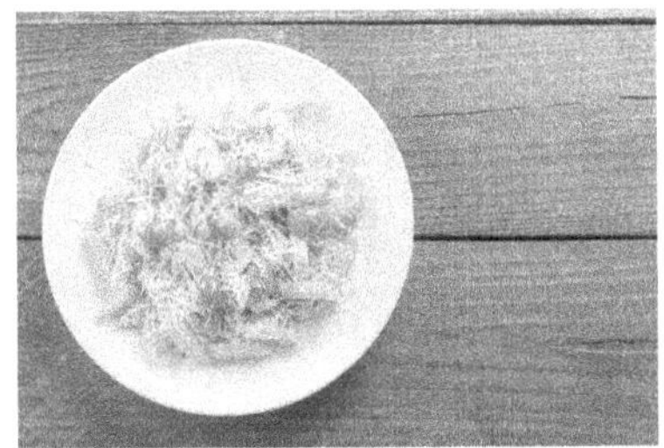

Ingredients:

- 1 medium spaghetti squash
- 2 tablespoons olive oil
- 1 cup marinara sauce (low-carb version)
- 1/4 cup fresh basil, chopped
- 1/4 cup grated Parmesan cheese (optional)
- Salt and pepper to taste

Instructions:

1. Preheat the oven to 400°F (200°C).
2. Cut the spaghetti squash in half lengthwise and scoop out the seeds.
3. Drizzle the inside with olive oil and season with salt and pepper.
4. Place the squash cut-side down on a baking sheet and roast for 40-45 minutes, until tender.
5. Once cooked, use a fork to scrape out the strands of squash.
6. Warm the marinara sauce in a pan over medium heat.

7. Toss the spaghetti squash with the marinara sauce and fresh basil.

8. Serve topped with grated Parmesan cheese if desired.

Nutritional Information (per serving, makes 4 servings):

- Calories: 150

- Protein: 5g

- Fat: 9g

- Carbohydrates: 14g

- Fiber: 3g

- Net Carbs: 11g

Slow Cooker Lentil Curry

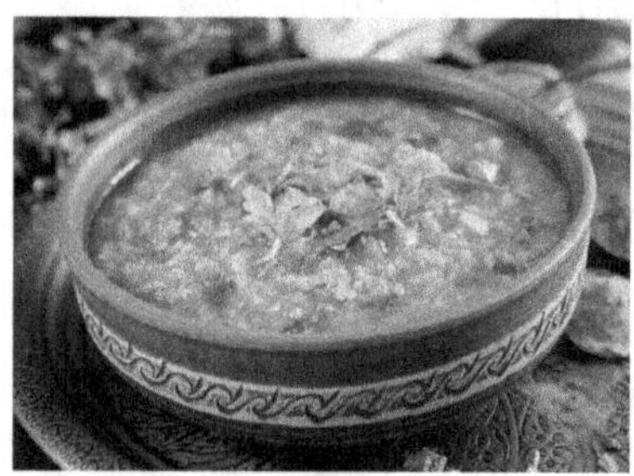

Ingredients:

- 1 cup dried green or brown lentils, rinsed
- 1 can (14.5 oz) diced tomatoes

- 1 cup vegetable broth
- 1 medium onion, diced
- 2 cloves garlic, minced
- 1 tablespoon curry powder
- 1 teaspoon ground cumin
- 1 teaspoon turmeric
- 1/2 teaspoon cayenne pepper (optional)
- 1 cup chopped spinach or kale
- Salt and pepper to taste

Instructions:

1. Place the lentils, diced tomatoes, vegetable broth, onion, garlic, curry powder, cumin, turmeric, and cayenne pepper into the slow cooker.
2. Stir to combine, cover, and cook on low for 6-8 hours or high for 3-4 hours, until the lentils are tender.
3. Stir in the spinach or kale in the last 30 minutes of cooking.
4. Adjust seasoning with salt and pepper before serving.

Nutritional Information (per serving, makes 6 servings):

- Calories: 220
- Protein: 13g
- Fat: 2g
- Carbohydrates: 38g
- Fiber: 13g
- Net Carbs: 25g

CHAPTER 11

Instant Pot Recipes

Beef Stew

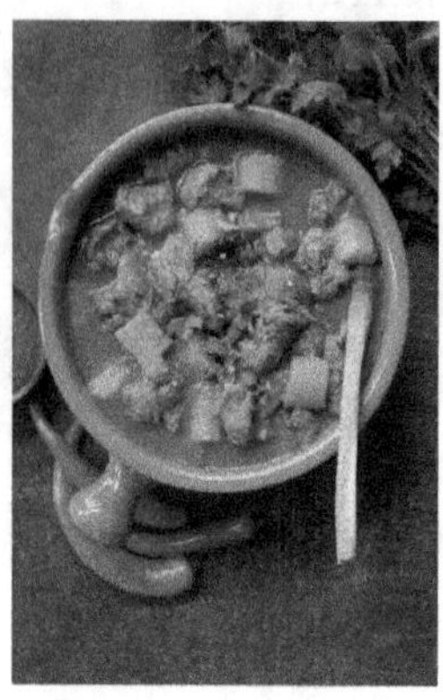

Ingredients:

- 2 lbs beef chuck, cut into cubes
- 2 tablespoons olive oil

- 1 large onion, diced
- 3 cloves garlic, minced
- 2 cups beef broth
- 1 cup red wine (optional)
- 2 cups carrots, sliced
- 1 cup celery, sliced
- 1 cup mushrooms, sliced
- 1 tablespoon tomato paste
- 1 teaspoon dried thyme
- 1 teaspoon dried rosemary
- 1 bay leaf
- Salt and pepper to taste

Instructions:

1. Set the Instant Pot to "Sauté" mode. Add olive oil and heat.
2. Add the beef cubes and brown on all sides. Remove and set aside.
3. Add the onion and garlic to the pot, cooking until softened.
4. Stir in the tomato paste, then return the beef to the pot.
5. Pour in the beef broth and red wine (if using), and add thyme, rosemary, bay leaf, salt, and pepper.

6. Close the lid and set the Instant Pot to "Manual" or "Pressure Cook" for 35 minutes.

7. After cooking, let the pressure release naturally.

8. Stir in the carrots, celery, and mushrooms. Set the pot to "Sauté" mode and cook for an additional 10-15 minutes, until vegetables are tender.

9. Remove the bay leaf before serving.

Nutritional Information (per serving, makes 6 servings):

- Calories: 340
- Protein: 30g
- Fat: 22g
- Carbohydrates: 10g
- Fiber: 2g
- Net Carbs: 8g

Chicken Tortilla-Less Soup

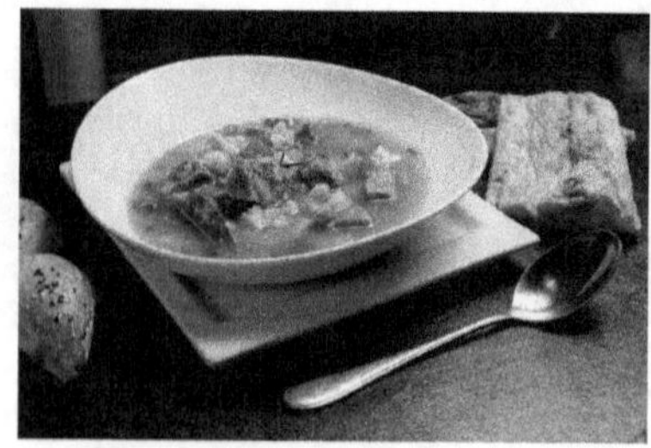

Ingredients:

- 1 lb chicken breasts or thighs
- 1 tablespoon olive oil
- 1 large onion, diced
- 2 cloves garlic, minced
- 1 bell pepper, diced
- 1 can (14.5 oz) diced tomatoes
- 1 cup chicken broth
- 1 cup corn kernels (optional)
- 1 teaspoon chili powder
- 1 teaspoon cumin
- 1/2 teaspoon paprika
- Salt and pepper to taste
- 1 cup shredded cheese (optional)
- Fresh cilantro for garnish (optional)

Instructions:

1. Set the Instant Pot to "Sauté" mode. Heat olive oil and add onion, garlic, and bell pepper. Cook until softened.
2. Add chicken breasts or thighs, diced tomatoes, chicken broth, corn (if using), chili powder, cumin, paprika, salt, and pepper.
3. Close the lid and set the Instant Pot to "Manual" or "Pressure Cook" for 10 minutes.
4. After cooking, let the pressure release naturally. Remove chicken and shred with two forks.
5. Return the shredded chicken to the pot and stir well.
6. Serve with shredded cheese and fresh cilantro if desired.

Nutritional Information (per serving, makes 6 servings):

- *Calories: 250*
- Protein: 30g
- Fat: 8g
- Carbohydrates: 15g
- Fiber: 3g
- Net Carbs: 12g

Low-Carb Yogurt

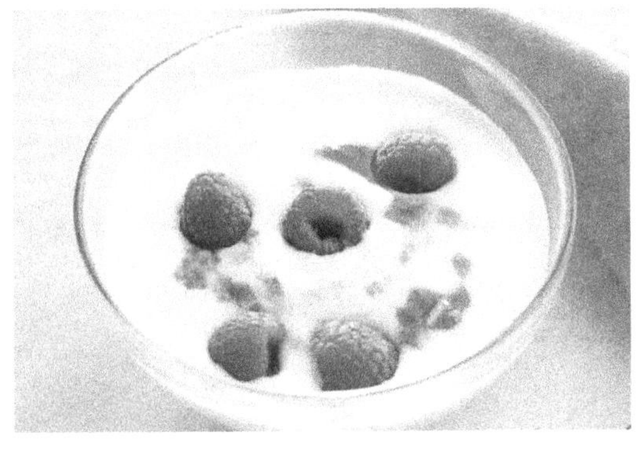

Ingredients:

- 4 cups unsweetened almond milk or coconut milk
- 2 tablespoons plain yogurt (for starter culture)
- 1/4 cup powdered erythritol or another low-carb sweetener (optional)

Instructions:

1. Pour almond milk or coconut milk into the Instant Pot and set to "Yogurt" mode. Heat until the milk reaches 180°F (82°C). Let cool to 110°F (43°C).
2. In a small bowl, mix the plain yogurt with a few tablespoons of cooled milk.

3. Stir the yogurt mixture back into the rest of the milk.

4. Set the Instant Pot to "Yogurt" mode again and incubate for 8-12 hours.

5. After incubation, transfer the yogurt to jars and refrigerate for at least 4 hours to thicken.

Nutritional Information (per serving, makes 6 servings):

- Calories: 50
- Protein: 2g
- Fat: 4g
- Carbohydrates: 2g
- Fiber: 0g
- Net Carbs: 2g

Ratatouille

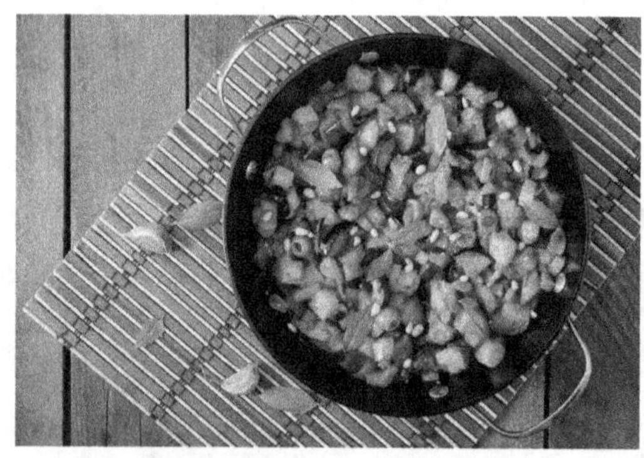

- 2 cloves garlic, minced
- 1 bell pepper, diced
- 1 zucchini, sliced
- 1 eggplant, diced
- 2 cups cherry tomatoes, halved
- 1 can (14.5 oz) diced tomatoes
- 1 teaspoon dried basil
- 1 teaspoon dried thyme
- Salt and pepper to taste

Ingredients:

- 2 tablespoons olive oil
- 1 large onion, diced

Instructions:

1. Set the Instant Pot to "Sauté" mode. Heat olive oil and add onion, garlic, and bell pepper. Cook until softened.
2. Add zucchini, eggplant, cherry tomatoes, diced tomatoes, basil, thyme, salt, and pepper.
3. Stir well and set the Instant Pot to "Manual" or "Pressure Cook" for 5 minutes.
4. After cooking, let the pressure release naturally.

Nutritional Information (per serving, makes 4 servings):

- Calories: 150
- Protein: 3g
- Fat: 10g
- Carbohydrates: 15g
- Fiber: 5g
- Net Carbs: 10g

Pulled Pork

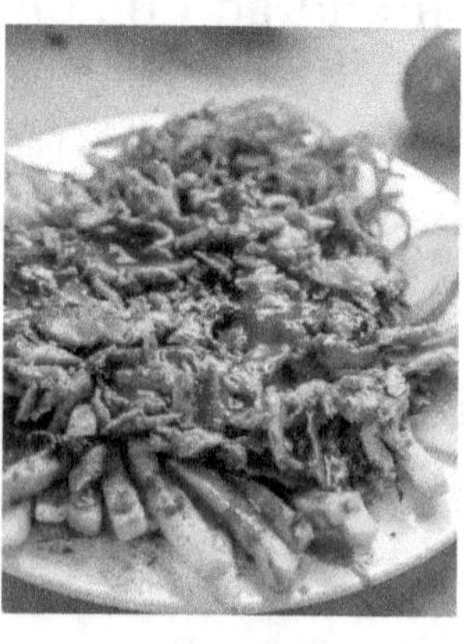

Ingredients:

- 3 lbs pork shoulder

- 1 tablespoon olive oil
- 1 large onion, diced
- 2 cloves garlic, minced
- 1 cup chicken broth
- 1/2 cup low-carb barbecue sauce
- 1 tablespoon paprika
- 1 tablespoon ground cumin
- 1 teaspoon dried oregano
- Salt and pepper to taste

Instructions:

1. Set the Instant Pot to "Sauté" mode. Heat olive oil and add onion and garlic. Cook until softened.
2. Season the pork shoulder with paprika, cumin, oregano, salt, and pepper.
3. Add the pork shoulder to the pot and brown on all sides.
4. Pour in the chicken broth and barbecue sauce.
5. Close the lid and set the Instant Pot to "Manual" or "Pressure Cook" for 60 minutes.
6. After cooking, let the pressure release naturally. Shred the pork with two forks and mix with the juices in the pot.
7. Serve as desired, with additional barbecue sauce if desired.

<u>Nutritional Information (per serving, makes 6 servings):</u>

- Calories: 350
- Protein: 30g
- Fat: 22g
- Carbohydrates: 10g
- Fiber: 1g
- Net Carbs: 9g

CHAPTER 12

Slow Cooker Recipes

<u>Pork Carnita</u>

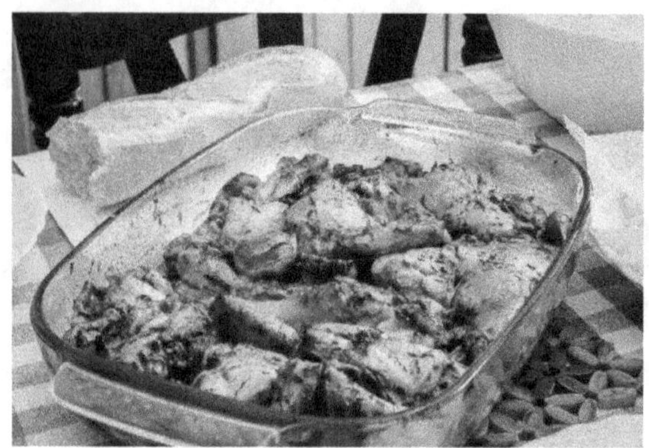

- 1 large onion, chopped
- 4 cloves garlic, minced
- 1/2 cup orange juice (or a low-carb alternative)
- 1/4 cup lime juice
- 1 tablespoon chili powder
- 1 teaspoon ground cumin
- 1 teaspoon dried oregano
- 1 teaspoon smoked paprika
- Salt and pepper to taste
- 2 bay leaves

<u>Ingredients:</u>

- 3 lbs pork shoulder, cut into chunks
- 1 tablespoon olive oil

<u>Instructions:</u>

1. Heat olive oil in a skillet over medium-high heat. Brown the pork chunks on all sides and transfer to the slow cooker.
2. Add the onion and garlic to the slow cooker.
3. Stir in the orange juice, lime juice, chili powder, cumin, oregano, paprika, salt, and pepper.
4. Add the bay leaves.
5. Cover and cook on low for 8-10 hours or on high for 4-5 hours, until the pork is tender.

6. Shred the pork with two forks and mix well with the juices.

7. Serve in tacos, bowls, or over a salad.

Nutritional Information (per serving, makes 6 servings):

- Calories: 350
- Protein: 30g
- Fat: 22g
- Carbohydrates: 8g
- Fiber: 1g
- Net Carbs: 7g

Creamy Chicken and Spinach

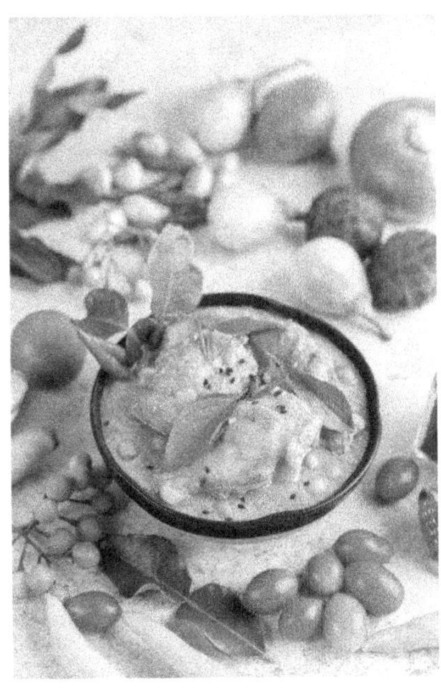

Ingredients:

- 4 boneless, skinless chicken breasts
- 1 can (14.5 oz) diced tomatoes
- 1 cup heavy cream
- 1 cup chicken broth
- 2 cups fresh spinach
- 1 tablespoon garlic powder
- 1 teaspoon dried basil
- 1 teaspoon dried oregano
- Salt and pepper to taste

Instructions:

1. Place the chicken breasts in the slow cooker.
2. In a bowl, mix together the diced tomatoes, heavy cream, chicken broth, garlic powder, basil, oregano, salt, and pepper.
3. Pour the mixture over the chicken breasts.
4. Cover and cook on low for 6-8 hours or on high for 3-4 hours, until the chicken is cooked through.
5. About 30 minutes before serving, stir in the fresh spinach and cook until wilted.
6. Shred the chicken and mix with the sauce before serving.

Nutritional Information (per serving, makes 4 servings):

- Calories: 380
- Protein: 32g
- Fat: 26g
- Carbohydrates: 6g
- Fiber: 2g
- Net Carbs: 4g

<u>Vegetable Medley</u>

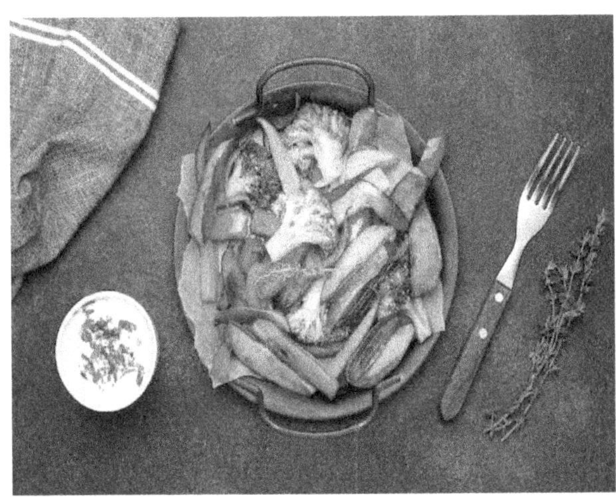

<u>Ingredients:</u>

- 2 cups carrots, sliced
- 2 cups green beans, trimmed
- 2 cups zucchini, sliced
- 1 cup bell peppers, diced
- 1 large onion, chopped
- 2 cloves garlic, minced
- 1/4 cup olive oil
- 1 teaspoon dried thyme
- 1 teaspoon dried rosemary
- Salt and pepper to taste

<u>Instructions:.</u>

1. Place all vegetables in the slow cooker.
2. In a bowl, mix together olive oil, garlic, thyme, rosemary, salt, and pepper.
3. Pour the olive oil mixture over the vegetables and toss to coat.
4. Cover and cook on low for 4-6 hours or on high for 2-3 hours, until vegetables are tender.
5. Serve warm.

<u>*Nutritional Information (per serving, makes 6 servings):*</u>

- Calories: 150
- Protein: 3g
- Fat: 9g
- Carbohydrates: 18g
- Fiber: 6g
- Net Carbs: 12g

Beef and Broccoli

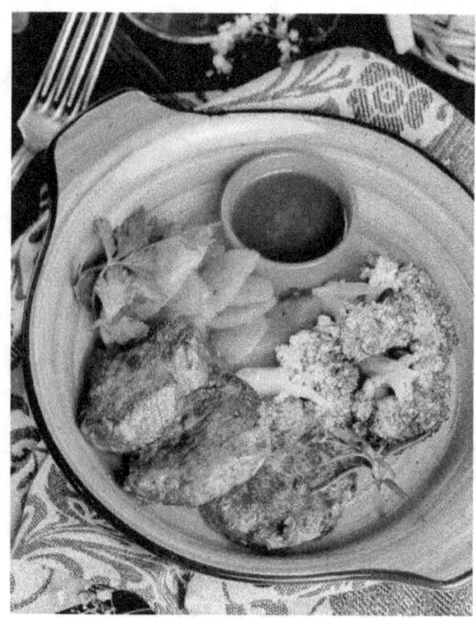

Ingredients:

- 1.5 lbs beef sirloin, sliced thinly
- 3 cups broccoli florets
- 1/2 cup soy sauce or tamari
- 1/4 cup beef broth
- 2 tablespoons hoisin sauce (check for low-carb version)
- 1 tablespoon cornstarch or xanthan gum (for thickening)
- 2 cloves garlic, minced
- 1 tablespoon sesame oil
- Salt and pepper to taste
- Sesame seeds for garnish (optional)

Instructions:

1. Place the beef slices in the slow cooker.
2. In a bowl, mix together soy sauce, beef broth, hoisin sauce, garlic, sesame oil, salt, and pepper.
3. Pour the mixture over the beef and toss to coat.
4. Cover and cook on low for 5-6 hours or on high for 3-4 hours, until beef is tender.
5. About 30 minutes before serving, stir in the broccoli florets.
6. If needed, mix cornstarch with a bit of water and stir into the sauce to thicken.
7. Garnish with sesame seeds if desired before serving.

Nutritional Information (per serving, makes 4 servings):

- Calories: 280
- Protein: 30g
- Fat: 14g
- Carbohydrates: 10g
- Fiber: 4g
- Net Carbs: 6g

Minestrone Soup

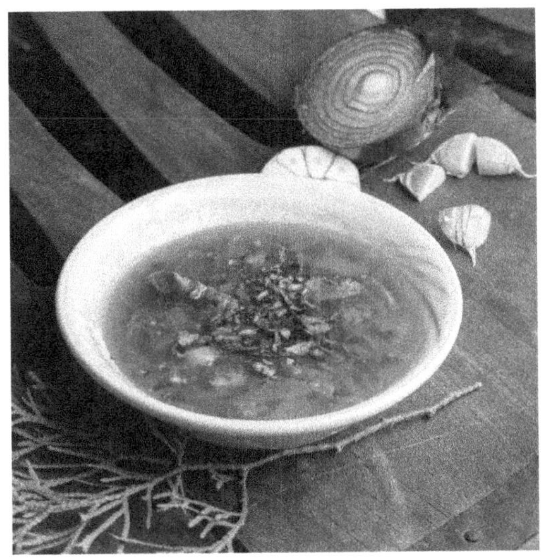

- 2 cups carrots, diced
- 2 cups celery, diced
- 1 can (14.5 oz) diced tomatoes
- 4 cups vegetable broth
- 1 cup green beans, chopped
- 1 cup zucchini, diced
- 1 cup spinach or kale
- 1 teaspoon dried basil
- 1 teaspoon dried oregano
- 1 bay leaf
- Salt and pepper to taste

Ingredients:

- 1 large onion, diced
- 2 cloves garlic, minced

Instructions:

1. Place the onion, garlic, carrots, and celery in the slow cooker.

2. Add the diced tomatoes, vegetable broth, green beans, zucchini, basil, oregano, bay leaf, salt, and pepper.
3. Stir to combine and cover.
4. Cook on low for 6-8 hours or on high for 3-4 hours.
5. Stir in the spinach or kale in the last 30 minutes of cooking.
6. Remove the bay leaf before serving.

Nutritional Information (per serving, makes 6 servings):

- Calories: 150
- Protein: 5g
- Fat: 5g
- Carbohydrates: 20g
- Fiber: 6g
- Net Carbs: 14g

CHAPTER 13

Staying on Track

Tips for Dining Out on a Low-Carb Diet

1. **Plan Ahead:** Many restaurants provide their menus online. Review the menu before going out to identify low-carb options.

2. **Choose Protein-Based Meals:** Opt for grilled or baked proteins like chicken, fish, or beef. Avoid breaded or fried options.

3. **Ask for Modifications:** Don't hesitate to request changes, such as substituting starchy sides with extra vegetables or requesting sauces on the side.

4. **Be Mindful of Sauces and Dressings:** Many sauces and dressings contain hidden sugars. Ask for them on the side and use them sparingly.

5. **Drink Smart:** Stick to water, unsweetened tea, or low-carb drinks. Avoid sugary cocktails and sodas.

Handling Social Situations and Holidays

1. **Communicate Your Needs:** Inform friends and family in advance about your dietary preferences. Offer to bring a low-carb dish to gatherings.

2. **Focus on the Sides:** At parties or dinners, fill up on salads, veggies, and protein-based dishes. Avoid high-carb appetizers like bread and pastries.

3. **Practice Portion Control:** If there are limited low-carb options, take smaller portions and savor them slowly.

4. **Stay Positive:** Emphasize the enjoyable aspects of socializing rather than focusing on food. Engaging in conversation and activities can help shift the focus away from eating.

Overcoming Plateaus

1. **Reevaluate Your Carb Intake:** Ensure you're staying within your target carb range. Sometimes a slight adjustment can help break a plateau.

2. **Track Your Progress:** Keep a food diary to monitor what you're eating and identify any potential issues.

3. **Increase Physical Activity:** Incorporate a mix of cardio, strength training, and flexibility exercises to boost metabolism.

4. **Change Up Your Routine:** Vary your diet and exercise routine to challenge your body in new ways. This can help overcome metabolic resistance.

Listening to Your Body and Making Adjustments

1. **Pay Attention to Hunger and Fullness:** Eat when you're hungry and stop when you're satisfied, not full. Adjust portion sizes based on your body's signals.

2. **Monitor Your Energy Levels:** If you're feeling unusually fatigued, it might be time to reassess your nutrient intake or meal timing.

3. **Evaluate Your Mood and Sleep:** Changes in mood or sleep patterns can indicate that your diet may need tweaking. Ensure you're getting balanced nutrition and enough rest.

4. **Consult a Professional:** If you're struggling despite your best efforts, consider consulting a dietitian or healthcare provider for personalized advice and support.

Frequently Asked Questions

Common Challenges and Solutions

1. Challenge: Finding Low-Carb Alternatives

- **Solution:** Explore low-carb substitutes for high-carb ingredients. For example, use zucchini or spaghetti squash in place of pasta, and almond or coconut flour instead of wheat flour. Many low-carb products are available in stores and online.

2. Challenge: Staying Full on a Low-Carb Diet

- **Solution:** Incorporate high-protein foods and healthy fats to keep you satisfied. Foods like avocados, nuts, seeds, and lean meats can help you feel full longer. Adding fiber-rich vegetables also supports satiety.

3. Challenge: Dealing with Cravings

- **Solution:** Choose low-carb snacks that satisfy cravings, such as cheese, nuts, or berries. Staying hydrated and eating balanced meals can also reduce cravings. If cravings persist, reassess your carb intake or nutrient balance.

4. Challenge: Eating Out and Social Situations

- **Solution:** Plan ahead by reviewing restaurant menus and making special requests. Focus on protein and vegetable dishes, and ask for dressings and sauces on the side. Bringing your own low-carb dishes to gatherings can also be helpful.

5. Challenge: Maintaining Variety in Meals

- **Solution:** Use a variety of herbs, spices, and cooking methods to keep meals interesting. Explore new recipes and try different low-carb ingredients to add variety to your diet.

FAQs About Low-Carb Cooking and Baking

1. Can I bake with low-carb ingredients?

- **Yes!** You can use almond flour, coconut flour, and other low-carb sweeteners like erythritol and stevia to bake delicious treats. Follow specific low-carb recipes for best results.

2. How can I make low-carb bread?

- **Low-carb bread recipes often use almond or coconut flour and eggs to replace traditional wheat flour.** Look for recipes that include these ingredients for a satisfying low-carb bread option.

3. Are there low-carb alternatives to rice and pasta?

- **Absolutely.** Cauliflower rice and zucchini noodles are excellent low-carb substitutes. You can also use spaghetti squash or konjac noodles as alternatives.

4. How can I thicken sauces without flour?

- **You can use xanthan gum, guar gum, or cornstarch in small amounts to thicken sauces.** Blending a portion of the dish to thicken it naturally is another effective method.

5. Can I use my regular cookware for low-carb recipes?

- **Yes,** you can use most of your regular cookware for low-carb recipes. Just be sure to follow the recipe instructions for best results and adjust cooking times as needed.

Nutritional Information for Low-Carb Dieters

1. How do I calculate net carbs?

- **Net carbs** are calculated by subtracting fiber and certain sugar alcohols (like erythritol) from the total carbohydrates. This helps you track carbs that impact blood sugar levels.

2. What's the recommended daily carb intake on a low-carb diet?

- **It varies,** but many low-carb diets recommend between 20-50 grams of net carbs per day. The exact amount can depend on your personal health goals and metabolic response.

3. Is it necessary to count calories on a low-carb diet?

- **Not necessarily.** While some people find counting calories helpful, many low-carb dieters focus more on carb intake and eat until they're full. Tracking calories can be useful if you have specific weight loss goals.

4. How do I get enough fiber on a low-carb diet?

- **Include high-fiber, low-carb vegetables such as leafy greens, broccoli, and cauliflower in your diet.** You can also use fiber supplements if needed to meet your daily requirements.

5. Can I have dairy on a low-carb diet?

- **Yes,** many low-carb diets include dairy products like cheese, yogurt, and butter. Opt for full-fat, unsweetened options to keep carbs low.

CONCLUSION

Establishing a Low Carb Lifestyle

Finally, it's important to revisit the profound benefits that this low carb diet can offer. By implementing a low-carb diet, many have experienced significant improvements in health markers, such as reduced blood sugar levels, better weight management, and enhanced energy levels. This approach not only helps in controlling hunger and cravings but also supports overall well-being through improved mental clarity and stable moods.

Recap of Benefits

The benefits of a low-carb diet extend far beyond simple weight loss. Reduced carbohydrate intake can lead to improved metabolic health, making it easier to manage conditions such as diabetes and insulin resistance. Many individuals find that they have more sustained energy throughout the day, as their bodies adapt to burning fat rather than sugar for fuel. Additionally, the increased intake of nutrient-dense, low-carb foods contributes to overall better health, with positive effects on cardiovascular health and reduced inflammation.

Encouragement and Final Tips

Transitioning to a low-carb lifestyle can initially seem challenging, but remember, it's a journey worth taking. Begin by setting realistic goals and celebrating small victories along the way. If you encounter obstacles or setbacks, don't be discouraged—every step you take towards healthier eating is a step in the right direction. Utilize the resources and tips provided in this book to make your transition smoother and more enjoyable.

Stay curious and open-minded as you explore new recipes and cooking techniques. Keep experimenting with different low-carb ingredients to discover what works best for you. It's also beneficial to stay connected with online communities or local groups that share your dietary goals, as they can offer support, share experiences, and provide additional inspiration.

Maintaining Your New Lifestyle

To successfully maintain your new low-carb lifestyle, incorporate it as part of your daily routine rather than viewing it as a temporary diet. Make meal planning and preparation a regular part of your week, and keep your kitchen stocked with essential low-carb ingredients. It's helpful to establish a balanced approach, allowing for occasional flexibility while staying focused on your core principles.

Remember, a low-carb lifestyle is not just about what you eat but also about how you approach your overall health and well-being. Embrace this lifestyle as a positive change rather than a restrictive diet, and take pride in the healthier choices you're making. By staying committed and proactive, you can enjoy the long-term benefits of a low-carb way of life, leading to a healthier, more vibrant you.

Glossary

Almond Flour: A low-carb alternative to wheat flour made from finely ground almonds. It's often used in baking and cooking to create low-carb bread, cakes, and other baked goods.

Banting Diet: A low-carb, high-fat diet named after William Banting. It emphasizes high-fat, low-carb foods while avoiding sugar, grains, and processed foods.

Bulletproof Coffee: A drink made with coffee, butter, and MCT oil (medium-chain triglycerides). It's popular in low-carb and ketogenic diets for its high fat content and energy-boosting effects.

Cauliflower Rice: Shredded or processed cauliflower that resembles rice in texture and appearance. It's used as a low-carb substitute for regular rice.

Erythritol: A sugar alcohol used as a low-carb sweetener. It has minimal calories and doesn't significantly affect blood sugar levels.

Fiber: The indigestible part of plant foods that helps with digestion and can aid in maintaining a healthy weight. On a low-carb diet, fiber is subtracted from total carbs to calculate net carbs.

Ketogenic Diet (Keto): A very low-carb, high-fat diet that aims to induce ketosis, a metabolic state where the body burns fat for fuel instead of carbohydrates.

Konjac Noodles: Also known as shirataki noodles, these are made from the konjac plant and are extremely low in carbs and calories. They're used as a substitute for traditional pasta.

Low-Carb Sweeteners: Sugar substitutes like stevia, monk fruit, and erythritol that provide sweetness without adding significant carbs or calories.

Net Carbs: The total carbohydrates in a food minus fiber and certain sugar alcohols (such as erythritol) that do not significantly affect blood sugar levels.

Paleo Diet: A diet based on consuming foods similar to those available to our pre-agricultural ancestors. It focuses on meat, fish, fruits, vegetables, nuts, and seeds while excluding processed foods, grains, and dairy.

Shirataki Noodles: Noodles made from the konjac root. They are very low in carbs and calories and are often used as a substitute for pasta in low-carb diets.

Xanthan Gum: A thickening agent made from fermented sugars. It's commonly used in low-carb cooking and baking to add texture and consistency to sauces and baked goods.

Zoodles: Noodles made from spiralized zucchini. They are a popular low-carb substitute for traditional pasta.

BONUS SECTION

PRINTABLE MEAL PLAN

One Week Low-Carb Meal Plan

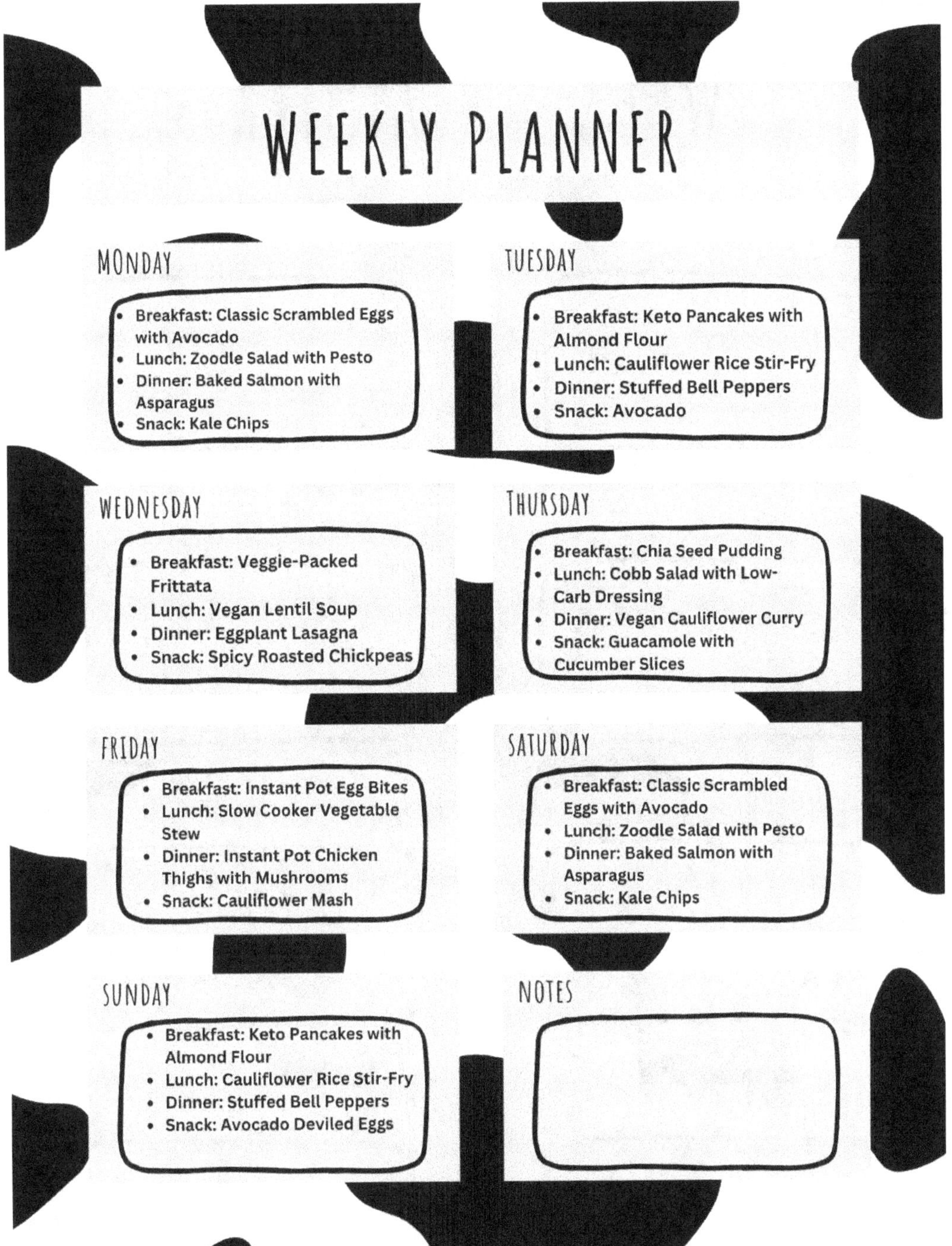

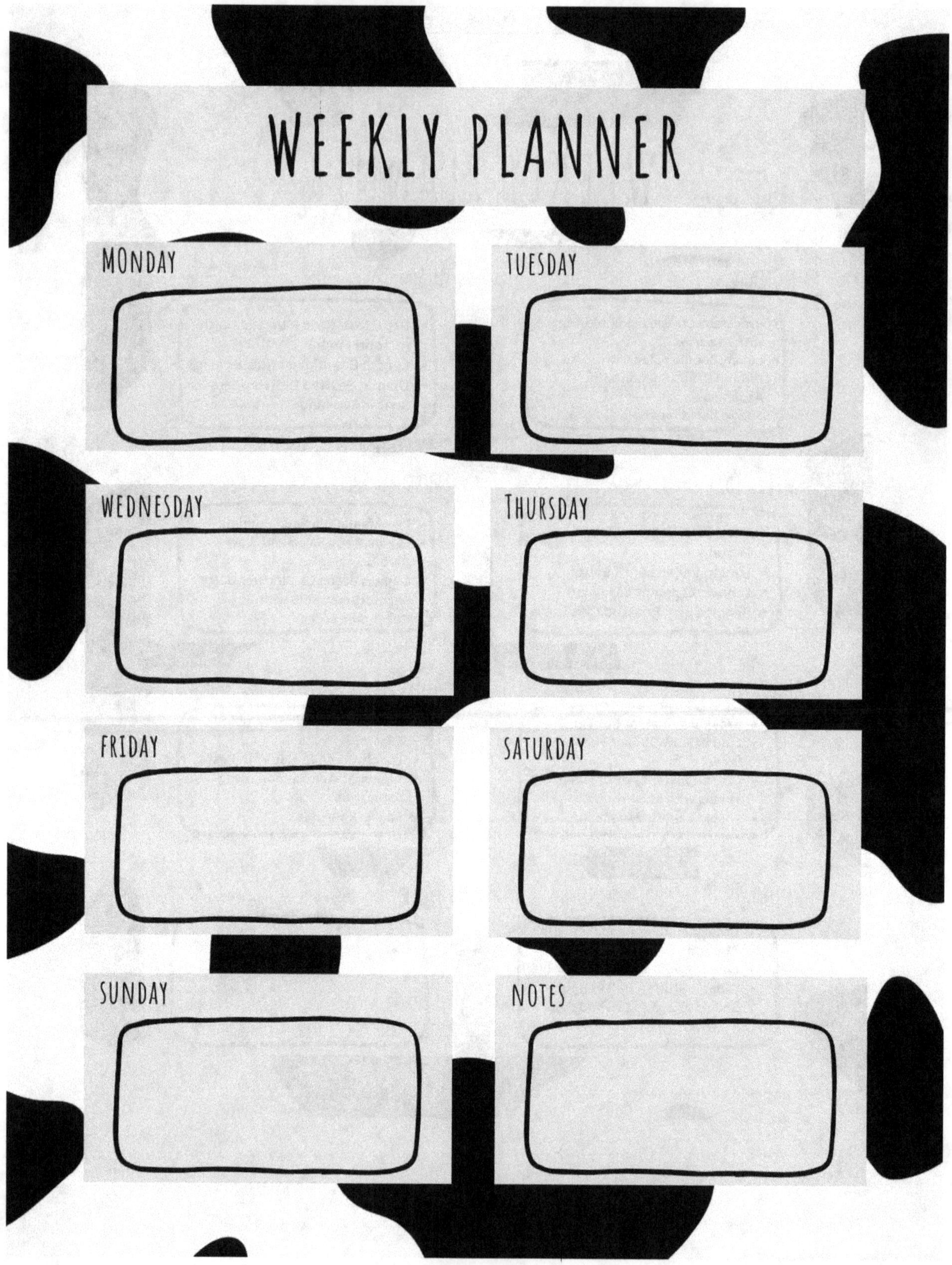
WEEKLY PLANNER
MONDAY
TUESDAY
WEDNESDAY
THURSDAY
FRIDAY
SATURDAY
SUNDAY
NOTES

<u>Shopping Lists For Each Week</u>

☐ **Proteins:** Eggs, salmon, chicken thighs, ground beef, tofu

☐ **Vegetables:** Avocado, zucchini, cauliflower, bell peppers, asparagus, kale, broccoli, spinach

☐ **Fruits:** Berries

☐ **Dairy:** Butter, heavy cream, almond milk, cheese

☐ **Pantry:** Almond flour, coconut flour, chia seeds, olive oil, coconut oil, nuts, seeds, spices (basil, oregano, thyme, rosemary, paprika, chili powder, cumin)

☐ **Condiments:** Low-carb salad dressing, pesto

☐ **Others:** Erythritol, stevia

MEAL PREP GUIDE

Sunday:

- Prepare Keto Pancakes and store in the fridge for quick breakfasts.
- Make a large batch of Chia Seed Pudding for breakfasts and snacks.
- Cook and store Classic Scrambled Eggs with Avocado for Monday and Tuesday breakfasts.
- Spiralize zucchini for Zoodle Salad and store in airtight containers.

- Prepare and marinate chicken thighs for Instant Pot Chicken Thighs with Mushrooms.
- Make Cauliflower Rice and store in the fridge.
- Chop and store vegetables (bell peppers, asparagus, kale, broccoli) for easy access.

Monday:

- Prepare a batch of Spicy Roasted Chickpeas for snacks throughout the week.
- Cook a large batch of Vegan Lentil Soup for lunches.

Wednesday:

- Make a big batch of Baked Salmon with Asparagus and store leftovers for future meals.
- Prepare Eggplant Lasagna and store in the fridge.

Friday:

- Prepare Slow Cooker Vegetable Stew for easy meals over the weekend.
- Cook Instant Pot Egg Bites for quick breakfasts or snacks.

By preparing meals and ingredients in advance, you'll save time during the week and make it easier to stick to your low-carb lifestyle. Adjust the meal plans and shopping lists based on your personal preferences and dietary needs for subsequent weeks.

Low Carb Diet Tips and Tricks

Practical Tips for Staying on Track with a Low-Carb Diet

1. **Keep It Simple:** Focus on whole, unprocessed foods. Stick to meats, fish, eggs, low-carb vegetables, nuts, and seeds.

   Simplify your meals with easy recipes that don't require complicated ingredients or cooking techniques.

2. **Prep Ahead:** Spend a couple of hours each week preparing meals and snacks. Chop vegetables, cook proteins, and portion out meals to make sticking to your diet easier during busy days.

   Use batch cooking to prepare large quantities of meals that can be stored and eaten throughout the week.

3. **Stay Hydrated:** Drink plenty of water throughout the day to stay hydrated and help curb cravings.

   Include beverages like herbal teas, black coffee, and water with lemon to add variety without adding carbs.

4. **Monitor Your Progress:** Keep a food diary to track what you eat and how it makes you feel. This can help identify foods that work best for you and keep you accountable.
   Use apps or online tools to track your carb intake and ensure you're staying within your target range.

5. **Have Go-To Snacks**: Keep low-carb snacks readily available to prevent reaching for high-carb options. Examples include cheese sticks, nuts, seeds, hard-boiled eggs, and low-carb vegetables like cucumber and bell pepper slices.

Strategies for Dining Out and Traveling

Research Before You Go:

Look up menus online before dining out to identify low-carb options and plan your meal in advance.

Choose restaurants known for offering healthy, customizable dishes, such as steakhouses, seafood restaurants, or places with salad bars.

Make Special Requests:

Don't be afraid to ask for modifications, such as replacing starchy sides with extra vegetables or requesting sauces on the side.

Most restaurants are accommodating if you explain your dietary needs politely.

Stick to Protein and Veggies:

Opt for dishes that are primarily composed of protein and vegetables. Grilled or baked meats, salads, and steamed or roasted veggies are typically good choices.

Avoid breaded or fried items, and skip the bread basket and sugary drinks.

Smart Travel Tips:

Pack your own low-carb snacks for the journey, such as nuts, cheese sticks, and sliced veggies, to avoid relying on convenience store options.

Research local grocery stores at your destination to stock up on essentials when you arrive.

Plan for Flexibility:

Allow some flexibility in your diet while traveling. If you indulge in a higher-carb meal, get back on track with your next meal.

Focus on making the best choices available without stressing over perfection.

Snack Ideas and Quick Fixes

- ❖ **Cheese and Meat Roll-Ups**: Roll slices of cheese and deli meat together for a quick, satisfying snack.
- ❖ **Vegetable Sticks with Dip:** Pair cucumber, bell pepper, and celery sticks with guacamole, hummus, or a low-carb dressing.

- ❖ **Boiled Eggs:** Hard-boiled eggs are an excellent high-protein, low-carb snack that can be prepared in advance.

Portable Snacks:

- ❖ **Nuts and Seeds**: Pack small portions of almonds, walnuts, or sunflower seeds for an easy, on-the-go snack.
- ❖ **Low-Carb Protein Bars:** Look for bars specifically designed to be low in carbs and high in protein.

Sweet Treats:

- ❖ **Berries and Cream**: Enjoy a small portion of fresh berries with a dollop of whipped cream.
- ❖ **Chia Seed Pudding**: Prepare chia seed pudding with unsweetened almond milk and a low-carb sweetener for a satisfying treat.

Quick Fix Meals:

- ❖ **Lettuce Wraps:** Use large lettuce leaves to wrap up your favorite proteins and vegetables for a quick, low-carb meal.
- ❖ **Tuna or Chicken Salad:** Mix canned tuna or chicken with mayonnaise and seasonings, then serve over a bed of greens or in a lettuce wrap.

By adopting these tips, strategies, and snack ideas as part of your daily routine, maintaining a low-carb lifestyle can be more manageable and enjoyable. Remember, the key to success is preparation, flexibility, and finding what works best for you.

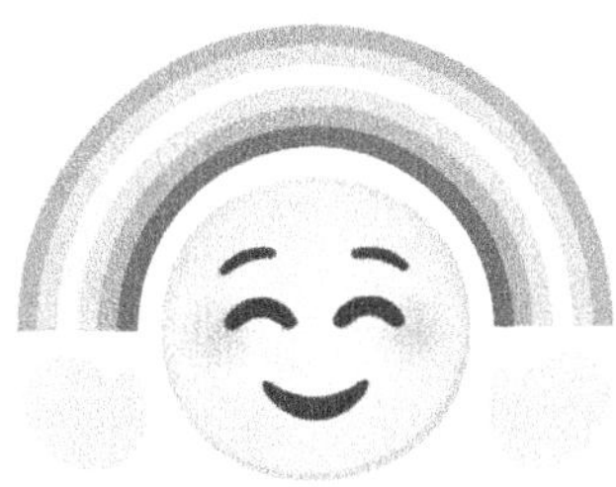

Thank you for reading 🙏